CONTENTS

Overview

Chapter One: Discrimination

Chapter Two: Learning Disabilities

Introduction

Disability Issues is the ninety-first volume in the **Issues** series. The aim of this series is to offer up-to-date information about important issues in our world.

Disability Issues looks at disability discrimination and learning disabilities.

The information comes from a wide variety of sources and includes:
Government reports and statistics
Newspaper reports and features
Magazine articles and surveys
Website material
Literature from lobby groups
and charitable organisations.

It is hoped that, as you read about the many aspects of the issues explored in this book, you will critically evaluate the information presented. It is important that you decide whether you are being presented with facts or opinions. Does the writer give a biased or an unbiased report? If an opinion is being expressed, do you agree with the writer?

Disability Issues offers a useful starting-point for those who need convenient access to information about the many issues involved. However, it is only a starting-point. At the back of the book is a list of organisations which you may want to contact for further information.

*****

Definition of disability

Information from the Disability Rights Commission

What counts as a disability according to the law?

The Disability Discrimination Act (DDA) protects disabled people. The Act sets out the circumstances in which a person is 'disabled'. It says you are disabled if you have:

- a mental or physical impairment
- this has an adverse effect on your ability to carry out normal day-to-day activities
- the adverse effect is substantial
- the adverse effect is long-term (meaning it has lasted for 12 months, or is likely to last for more than 12 months or for the rest of your life).

There are some special provisions, for example:

- if your disability has badly affected your ability to carry out normal day-to-day activities, but doesn't any more, it will still be counted as having that effect if it is likely to do so again
- if you have a progressive condition such as HIV or multiple sclerosis or arthritis, and it will badly affect your ability to carry out normal day-to-day activities in the future, it will be treated as having a bad effect on you now
- past disabilities are covered.

What are 'normal day-to-day activities'?

At least one of these areas must be badly affected:

- mobility
- manual dexterity
- physical co-ordination
- continence
- ability to lift, carry or move everyday objects
- speech, hearing or eyesight
- memory or ability to concentrate, learn or understand
- understanding of the risk of physical danger.

 Disability Rights Commission

It's really important to think about the effect of your disability without treatment. The Act says that any treatment or correction should not be taken into account, including medical treatment or the use of a prosthesis or other aid (for example, a hearing aid). The only things which are taken into account are glasses or contact lenses.

The important thing is to work out exactly how your disability affects you. Remember to concentrate on what you can't do, or find difficult, rather than what you can do.

For example, if you have a hearing disability, being unable to hold a conversation with someone talking normally in a moderately noisy place would be a bad effect. Being unable to hold a conversation in a very noisy place such as a factory floor would not.

If your disability affects your mobility, being unable to travel a short journey as a passenger in a vehicle would be a bad effect. So would only being able to walk slowly or with unsteady or jerky movements. But having difficulty walking without help for about 1.5 kilometres or a mile without having to stop would not.

What does not count as a disability?

Certain conditions are not considered impairments under the DDA:

- lifestyle choices such as tattoos and non-medical piercings
- tendency to steal, set fires, and physical or sexual abuse of others
- exhibitionism and voyeurism
- hayfever, if it doesn't aggravate the effects of an existing condition
- addiction to or a dependency on alcohol, nicotine or any other substance, other than the substance being medically prescribed.

■ The above information is from the Disability Rights Commission's website which can be found at www.drc-gb.org

© 2004 Disability Rights Commission (DRC)

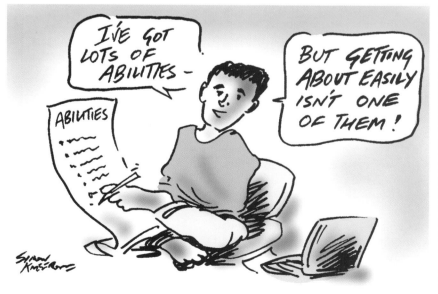

I'VE GOT LOTS OF ABILITIES –

BUT GETTING ABOUT EASILY ISN'T ONE OF THEM!

ABILITIES

Public attitudes to disabilities

A YouGov survey for Scope

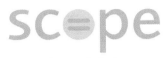

About cerebral palsy.
For disabled people achieving equality.

Introduction

Scope commissioned YouGov to assess public attitudes to disability and disabled people. The survey was conducted among a representative sample of 2,151 adults online throughout Great Britain between 7 and 11 May 2004.

Because disability is a term that covers a wide range of impairments, a questionnaire was drawn up that not only explored general attitudes but also asked respondents how they would react to specific scenarios involving disabled people. In some cases, 'it depends' was offered as an answer-option. A randomly selected sub-group of respondents answering 'it depends' was then asked to state in their own words what it depended on.

Overall attitudes to disabled people and their rights

In general, the attitudes of the British public towards disability and disabled people are broadly positive and supportive.

87% believe that disabled people should have equal rights with non-disabled people; just 1% disagree; but 11% say 'it depends'.

These figures are much the same for each demographic group – by age, gender, social class and British region.

86% think a child with Down's Syndrome who needed a heart and lung transplant should be given an equal place with other children on the waiting list; a further 3% think the Down's Syndrome child should be treated earlier. Just 8% think the Down's Syndrome child should be treated later (7%) or not at all (1%).

80% think it is fair for disabled students to receive extra help when sitting an exam; just 7% say this is not fair.

40% think there are not enough disabled people on television. Only 1% think there are too many. 27% say there are enough, while a large proportion, 31%, have no opinion.

Men are equally divided between those who say 'enough' and 'not enough'. Among women a majority of more than two to one say 'not enough'.

Three out of four (76%) say it is acceptable for non-disabled people to play the part of a disabled person in a drama or film. Just 13% say this is not acceptable.

93% support the principle of disabled people having designated parking spaces; 6% admit to having parked in such a space without a permit.

Concerns

Despite overwhelming public support for equal rights, there are some circumstances in which a significant minority admit concern about the presence of disabled people.

More than one person in four said they would be concerned if:

- They discovered that a new football referee for their local league was deaf (31%)
- They discovered that their boss at work had dyslexia (29%)
- Their 19-year-old daughter

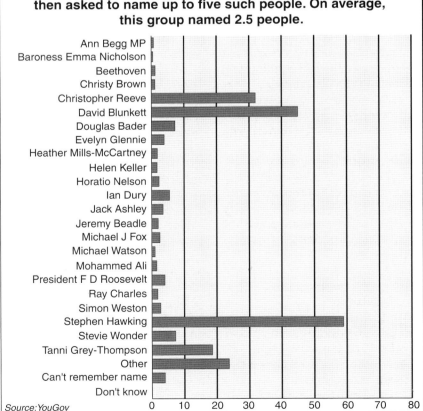

Knowledge of famous disabled people

Respondents were asked if they could name any famous disabled people. Almost two-thirds (64%) said they could. This group was then asked to name up to five such people. On average, this group named 2.5 people.

Source: YouGov

brought home a boyfriend who was disabled (28%)

- A local solicitor from whom they sought advice was blind (27%)
- At the other end of the scale, more than 85% said they would NOT be concerned if:
- They visited their local surgery and had to be seen by a locum wearing a hearing aid (98%)
- One of the children in their child's class at school was disabled (92%)
- Their child's teacher used a wheelchair (90%)
- They discovered, when going for a job interviewer, that the person making the final decision had cerebral palsy (87%)
- A company applied for planning permission to build accessible accommodation nearby for disabled people (87%)
- They noticed, when appearing in court on a speeding offence, that the magistrate used a communication aid to speak (87%)

'It depends'

The four issues that provoked the largest proportion of 'it depends' responses were:

1. If the respondent met someone through a dating agency and, after a series of telephone calls, discovered at their first face-to-face meeting that they were disabled (49%) – bringing the total saying they would change their mind or 'it depends' to 57%

Those who replied 'it depends' were then asked to say, in their own words, on what it depended. Two-thirds responded with some variant of 'the nature' or 'the extent' of the disability. Others said it depended on how well they got on when they met, or on the reasons given for concealing the disability beforehand.

Dating a disabled person – on what does it depend?

'Whether or not I found them attractive; there are disabled people who I do find attractive but if they looked like a pig then I wouldn't go out with them again.'

'How bad the disablement is, physical intimacy is also important.'

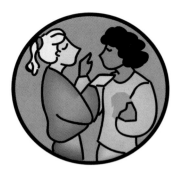

'On the reasons as to why the person has not previously mentioned the disability. This is a tricky one though, as it is a bit like meeting someone and then finding out they hadn't told you about e.g. they have children.'

'Core, common interests and my ability to cope with/manage and support their disability.'

2. Whether disabled people should receive benefits to pay for the extra costs of disability (40%). Once again, two thirds of these mentioned the severity of the disability. Significant numbers mentioned the need to relate benefits to costs and/ or to the person's ability to pay (including ability to work).

3. If their 19-year-old daughter brought home a disabled boyfriend (38%), bringing the total saying 'concerned' or 'it depends' to 66%.

4. Whether disabled people should have an equal right to become parents as non-disabled people (34%). In this case half of this group mentioned the severity of the disability, while two in five mentioned care issues and one in four mentioned fears of disabilities being inherited.

Rights for disabled people who wish to be parents – on what does it depend?

'On the severity of disability and the risk of that disability – if severe – being passed on to their children.'

That right should not extend to medical treatment in order to able to father/mother the child if the disability means they cannot already. That right should be limited if it can be proven the child is very likely to be born severely (acute and chronic) disabled.

How well they are physically, mentally and emotionally able to care for the child. Will they be able to

look after a small child properly? Will they have adequate help and support in doing so?

Paying to ensure that disabled people can exercise their rights

Half the public (52%) say they would 'definitely' go ahead with a holiday booking if their tour operator told them that a large group of disabled people would be staying at their hotel. A further 34% would 'probably' go ahead. 13% would either 'probably' or 'definitely' not go ahead.

22% would be prepared to pay 5% extra for their holiday to ensure that disabled people could enjoy the same kind of break. A further 30% would be prepared to pay 2% extra. However, 39% would not be prepared to pay extra.

Greatest resistance to paying extra is among those aged 30-50 – the people that take their children on holiday. 45% would not pay any extra.

There is greater public resistance to paying £15 a month extra on their council tax to make sure that all public transport in the area is accessible to disabled people. 20% support this, but 63% are opposed.

The public is evenly divided on whether a disabled person is likely to take more time off work than a non-disabled person, due to sickness or medical appointments.

By 48-30%, the public rejects the view that it could cost a lot extra for an employer to employ a disabled person.

Knowledge of famous disabled people

Respondents were asked if they could name any famous disabled people. Almost two-thirds (64%) said they could.

This group was then asked to name up to five such people. On average, this group named 2.5 people. The most frequently mentioned names were: Stephen Hawking (59%), David Blunkett (45%) and Christopher Reeve (32%).

The gender gap

Men are slightly more likely than women to express concern on most issues. The gender gap is widest on the following issues:

- Whether people feel uncomfortable being served in a clothes shop by someone with a facial disfigurement. 20% of men, but only 10% of women, say they would feel uncomfortable.

- Hiring a deaf referee for a local football league. 38% of men, but just 25% of women, would be concerned.
- Having a new work colleague who has dyslexia. 33% of men would have concerns, compared with 25% of women.
- A 19-year-old daughter having a disabled boyfriend. 32% of men would have concerns, compared with 27% of women. (By 44% to 32%, women are more likely than men to say 'it depends'.)
- By 47-33%, men think disabled workers are prone to take more time off; but by 43-33% women disagree.
- Men are fairly evenly divided on whether 'it could cost a lot extra to employ a disabled person in your workplace'; 36% think it could, while 45% think it would not. By women reject the proposition by two to one (51-24%)

Extra benefits for disabled people – on what does it depend?

'The level of support required. It is perfectly reasonable to pay an allowance to cover some extra transport costs etc., but there is a financial limit to how much extra support the taxpayer can provide, even though it may well be merited.'

'On the disability. But in most cases the councils or local governments are funded enough to cover these overheads.'

'If the disability prevents the person from working, or could measurably be proven to restrict the person's earning capability. I have asthma, but I have to pay for my medication still, I don't expect others to subsidise me for this though as I can earn money fine. Everyone has things they have to pay extra for in life.'

■ The above information is from a YouGov survey which was conducted for Scope. For further information about Scope's work visit their website: www.scope.org.uk

©YouGov

Disability

More boys than girls with disability

Slightly higher proportions of boys (19 per cent) than girls (17 per cent) aged under 20 years reported having a mild disability in 2000. Rates of severe disability were consistently higher for boys than girls with 11 per 10,000 of the male population and five per 10,000 of the female population aged under 17 years in 2000.

The most common condition reported among under 20-year-olds with a longstanding illness or disability was asthma with 42 per cent of total impairments in 2000. From 1990 to 1998, mental handicap (a term used by Family Fund Trust) was the predominant disability condition among severely disabled children and adolescents. In 1999 and 2000 the predominant disability conditions among severely disabled children and adolescents were autistic spectrum disorders and behavioural disorders.

The distribution of children and adolescents with mild disabilities was higher for those from semi-skilled manual and unskilled manual backgrounds. The highest prevalence rates of severe disability in children and adolescents were among those from semi-skilled manual backgrounds.

Disabled children and adolescents (37 per cent) were more likely to participate in swimming in school than the general population (30 per cent). Swimming was also the most popular sporting activity undertaken by disabled children and adolescents out of school. Horseriding was another sporting activity more frequently participated in, during school time, by disabled children and adolescents (six per cent) than the general population of young people (one per cent).

In 2001, disabled children and adolescents cited lack of money (37 per cent) and unsuitability of local sports facilities (37 per cent) as some of the reasons for experiencing difficulties in accessing leisure facilities out of school.

■ Mild disability is the term used to represent longstanding illness and disability referred to in the General Household Survey.

© Crown copyright

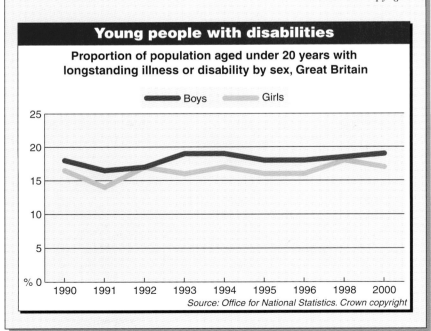

Young people with disabilities

Proportion of population aged under 20 years with longstanding illness or disability by sex, Great Britain

— Boys — Girls

Source: Office for National Statistics. Crown copyright

World of their own?

We often hear the term 'disabled community'. So what does the term mean? Who uses it? And who does it refer to? Some say it exists and indeed thrives, while others are adamant that it is nothing more than a convenient label. One topic, several points of view . . .

Just like we do not share a common religion, political belief or social class, disabled people do not share a common disability. While I do not deny my impairment in any way, I do reject an identity based on that impairment. There is now a widespread use of convenient labels throughout society, such as "the homeless" and "refugees", none of which adequately explain the individual circumstances or experiences.'

Maulani Rotinsulu, Chairman, Persatuan Penyandang Cacat Indonesia (Indonesian Disabled People Association)

'Disabled people make up between 10 and 20 per cent of the UK population and can have a wide range of impairments. But while many would not wish to be identified as part of a "disabled community", the advantage of disabled people meeting to share their experiences plays a valuable role in their empowerment and encourages them to take a more proactive role in wider society. Not everyone would want to be described as a part of it. But it is important to recognise the sociological role of such groups, like the black and feminist movements before it, based on a shared commitment to push for the full human and civil rights of disabled people.'

Clare Evans, Manager, Leonard Cheshire's Disabled People's Forum, United Kingdom

'While the importance of such a collective voice should not be overlooked, disability is a very individual and personal experience. It is something which can affect people of any age, sexuality, gender or religion. While people with a certain type of disability may identify with each other, very few are

committed to a wider programme of radical social change.'

Abdus Sattar Dulal, Executive Director and Founder, Bangladesh Protibandhi Kallyan Somity (Welfare Association for Persons with Disabilities in Bangladesh)

'Disabled people account for around 20 per cent of the Australian population and while they all share a common thread, people from such a diverse and multi-cultural society will experience disability in many different ways. While in general Australia is a community of activists and advocates, they still face a variety of issues and barriers to their acceptance into general society. It is therefore vital that we maintain strong political campaigns for their full independent access to mainstream society. The question of whether people identify as part of a national or international disabled community can't be answered yet and will remain so until a United Nations Convention [on the Rights of Disabled People] provides adequate time and access to address the issues which surround it.'

Rob Lake, Senior Policy Officer, People with Disability, Australia

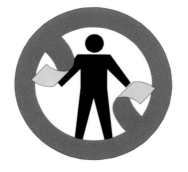

'I am a disabled person and when I use the word "disabled" about myself, I am making a statement. I have an impairment but my disability arises from the discrimination I endure as a result of society's failure to take full account of my rights and creates barriers to my full inclusion. Like a residential neighbourhood, disabled people find themselves together by virtue of being in a common place – in this case that "place" is a common experience of our rights being ignored and barriers encountered which deny our full social inclusion. Furthermore, like a neighbourhood, some members of the "disabled community" want to be part of that community life, while others don't. Those that do, deliberately seek out and identify with other disabled people because they benefit from each other's company – whether in political campaigning, the arts, sport or other fields of activity. While many recognise the need for organisations representing disabled people, the term "disabled community" implies segregation whereas we are working towards inclusion. If you were to define people by abilities and disabilities alone, then people would belong to a number of communities.'

Andy Rickell, Director, British Council of Disabled People, United Kingdom

■ Do you have any views on the subject? If so, we would like to hear your opinions and experiences. Please write to:

The Editor, *Compass*, Leonard Cheshire, 30 Millbank, London SW1P 4QD. Email: compass@lc-uk.org

■ The above information is from the Leonard Cheshire magazine *Compass*. For more information visit their website which can be found at www.leonard-cheshire.org

Disability issues

Information from Scope

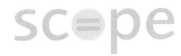

About cerebral palsy.
For disabled people achieving equality.

Background

Numbers of disabled people

We cannot be certain about the number of disabled people in Great Britain, as there is a range of different statistics. The main reasons for the variations are due to when and how the information was collected. For example, did people complete a questionnaire themselves, or did someone else decide whether they 'counted' as disabled?

According to the 2001 census results[1] there are 10.8 million people (of all ages) in the UK who have a long-term health problem or disability, which limits their daily activities or the work they could do. They make up 18.5% of the population.

Government research[2] estimates that there are 8.6 million disabled adults (aged 16+) living in private households in the UK (i.e. 20% of the adult population) and nearly 400,000 disabled children under the age of 16. This accounts for approximately one in 38 of all children in the population.[3]

The total number is likely to rise further with an increasingly elderly population, as the likelihood of disability increases with age.

Discrimination and attitudes

Disabled people continue to face discrimination and difficulties imposed by society in every area of their lives. The common experiences of disabled people are of rejection and enormous difficulty in taking part in even the most ordinary activities such as shopping, going to the cinema or to the pub.

Discrimination is present in education and employment, often leading to lifelong dependence on welfare benefits.

Many polling stations are inaccessible; therefore disabled people are denied the right to vote on equal terms with non-disabled people. In addition, disabled people are forced into dependence, suffer humiliation and struggle with an inaccessible environment every day.

As a consequence, many disabled people give up the struggle of attempting to take part in society and stay at home.

The exclusion of disabled people from society means that some non-disabled people have never met a disabled person and therefore do not have the opportunity to develop opinions and attitudes about them based on personal experience.

Lack of awareness and fear of the unknown is compounded by the predominantly negative media images of disabled people and of disability generally. For example, in a survey conducted by The Leonard Cheshire Foundation[4], nearly one-third of people questioned thought that wheelchair-users were 'less intelligent'; and 44% of opinion leaders thought that using a wheelchair would present a major obstacle to gaining employment. Such misconceptions lead to a vicious circle of rejection, discrimination and exclusion.

Language

What we say both reflects and shapes the way we think. The language we use about disability is an important way of influencing our own and society's attitudes.

Words and phrases to avoid include: handicapped person, spastic, wheelchair-bound, sufferer, the disabled.

Use the following instead: disabled person, has cerebral palsy, wheelchair-user, has an impairment.

Social versus medical model of disability

Behaviour towards disabled people is governed by the picture or 'model' of disability that others carry in their minds. These models, in turn, affect the way in which society is organised. The two main models are:

The medical model sees disability as an illness and disabled people as patients in need of a cure so that they can fit into 'normal' society. The emphasis is on the condition rather than the person.

The social model recognises disabled people as equals who are battling against very unequal odds i.e. society's attitudes. The emphasis is on society's responsibilities and changing attitudes rather than the disabled person's problem.

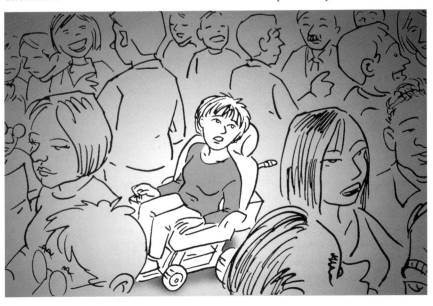

Education/inclusion

Discrimination against disabled people begins from the moment they are born. Disabled children are often segregated, mainly because of medical considerations, which undermines the possibility of enjoying life alongside non-disabled peers. However, the Special Educational Needs and Disability Act 2001 makes it unlawful for all education providers to discriminate against disabled pupils. Full details of these measures are available on the Disability Rights Commission website: www.drc.org.uk

Early school experiences (positive or negative) can have a profound impact on how disabled people feel about themselves and influence expectations about their future role in society.

Meanwhile, the controversy over special schools continues. Some people argue that whilst special segregated education exists, most non-disabled children will never come into contact with disabled children. Their attitudes therefore are formed from those of adults and the media, which often perpetuates negative attitudes and stereotyping. Disabled and non-disabled children learning and growing up together takes away the fear of the unknown and makes disability part of the norm.

98.9% of all children are educated in mainstream schools.

Around 1.4 million children (16.9% of pupils) in schools in England are identified as having Special Educational Needs (SEN). Primary schools have a slightly higher proportion (20.7%) than secondary schools (18.3%).

From 1997 to 2002 the total number of pupils in special schools fell from 98,200 to 94,500 and the total number of special schools fell by 6% to 1,161 across the UK, thus underlining the trend towards greater inclusion of disabled pupils.

The number of children with SEN Statements continues to rise with an increase of 11% in the last five years. However, there are wide variations within and between regions.

Of pupils with SEN Statements 60% are now educated in maintained mainstream schools (a rise from 48% since 1993), 37% in special schools (maintained and non-maintained) or Pupil Referral Units, and 3% in independent schools.

Employment

Many employers still favour non-disabled job applicants over disabled ones. This happens for a variety of reasons ranging from fear or prejudice to misunderstandings about people's abilities or the supposed costs of employing a disabled person.

Whilst some major companies are practising equal opportunities there are still instances of prejudice towards disabled colleagues among other employers or fellow employees. Once in employment disabled people do not always have the same promotion prospects as non-disabled colleagues and they may have to work harder to maintain their position within the organisation.

Of those looking for work, disabled people made an average of two and a half times as many job applications as non-disabled people and yet got fewer job offers

---

Disabled people account for almost 20% of the working-age population (6.8 million) and yet almost half of all disabled people of working age do not have a job.[5]

80.7% of non-disabled people are in employment compared with 48.9% of disabled people.[6]

There are one million disabled people who want to work but do not have a job.[7]

Of those looking for work, disabled people made an average of two and a half times as many job applications as non-disabled people and yet got fewer job offers.[8]

40% of employers, responding to the research, did not know if their premises would be accessible to someone with a physical impairment and 51% didn't know if disabled people applied for jobs with their company.[9]

Goods and services

In Scope's *Disabled In Britain* report one in three disabled people said they had been refused service in a public place such as cinema, restaurant, pub/club, theatre, sporting event or leisure centre. The Disability Discrimination Act (see below) has acted as a catalyst for commercial and public sector providers of goods and services to improve physical access as part of their service to disabled people as reported in Scope's research report, *In Good Company?*.[11]

Scope's *Left Out* report[12] showed that three-quarters of businesses had one or more entry problems for disabled people, and that nearly one-fifth of staff were not respectful to disabled customers.

Families/carers

In 1995, Scope published the results of its study into carers' lives – one of the largest studies ever undertaken – in *Disabled in Britain: behind closed doors – the carers' experience*.[13]

The needs of individual families and carers differ widely. This partly reflects the type of support available to them, and partly the needs of the person for whom they care (ranging from young carers and young disabled children, to elderly carers and elderly relatives being cared for). In this article, we are only able to give a partial picture of the needs of some families/carers.

Emotional/psychological needs

Carers, whether family, friends or employees, play a crucial role in the lives of disabled people. As well as being a potentially rewarding and satisfying role, caring for disabled people can be stressful and is often undervalued,[14] in both economic and status terms.

Caring for a disabled person also affects other members of the family, especially siblings. Parents may feel guilty about not giving enough time to siblings, and siblings may also harbour feelings of resentment about this. Three-quarters of respondents in Scope's 1995 survey[15] who cared for disabled children aged between 6 and 15 felt they sometimes neglected other family members, as opposed to 50% who cared for someone aged 65 or more.

Physical needs

Caring for a disabled person can be hard work. Many carers feel both physically tired and mentally fatigued because of the effort involved in obtaining and providing the services needed. Carers often put their own health and safety at risk through physical activity necessitated by lack of equipment, or through the mental worries brought about by the constant anxiety.

Financial/economic needs

'Caring costs', said Scope's 1995 report on caring.[16] It found that many respondents bear the bulk of the costs themselves: their careers suffer; they experience financial hardship and are frequently stressed and unwell.

Legislation

The Disability Discrimination Act 1995 (DDA) was passed in 1995 to introduce new measures aimed at ending discrimination against disabled people. Part 1 of the Act provides a definition of disability and sets out who is covered by the legislation. The Act aims to protect disabled people in the following areas:

- employment access to goods, facilities and services
- the management, buying or renting of land or property
- education

Some of these measures became law in 1996; others will be introduced over time.

Goods and services

Since December 1996, it has been unlawful for service providers and those responsible for selling, letting or managing premises:

- to refuse service
- to provide a worse standard of service
- to offer a service on worse terms to disabled people.

Since October 1999, further provisions have required service providers to make reasonable steps to:

a) Amend policies, procedures and practices that make it impossible

---

As well as being a potentially rewarding and satisfying role, caring for disabled people can be stressful and is often undervalued, in both economic and status terms

---

or unreasonably difficult for disabled people to access the service (e.g. a 'no dogs' policy in cases where visually impaired people wish to enter the premises with a guide dog).

b) Provide auxiliary aids and services where this would enable or facilitate disabled people's use of a service (e.g. lifting items off shelves in shops for those unable to manage alone).

c) Overcome physical features which make it impossible or unreasonably difficult for disabled people to use a service, by providing that service by a reasonable alternative method.

From 2004, service providers will have to:

- amend or remove physical feature(s) of the premises, which make it impossible or unreasonably difficult for disabled people to use a service, or provide a reasonable means of avoiding it.

Education

For education providers, new duties came into effect in September 2002 – details as above.

Transport

The DDA allows Government to set minimum standards to assist disabled people to use public transport easily. This will be phased in over a period of time.

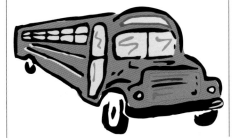

Disability Rights Commission (DRC)

The Disability Rights Commission (DRC) is an independent body, established by Act of Parliament, which aims to eliminate discrimination against disabled people and promote equality of opportunity.

It started work in April 2000 and undertakes formal investigations, carries out research and advises the Government on the operation and/or modification of the DDA. It also provides an advice and information service for disabled people, employers and service providers and campaigns to strengthen the law. For full details of their services visit their website at www.drc.org.uk

References and further reading
1. Census 2001 results at: www.statistics.gov.uk/census2001
2. Grundy et al. *Disability in Great Britain*. DSS/Corporate Document Services, 1999
3. *Quality Protects: Disabled Children, Numbers and Categories.* Department of Health, 2000
4. Knight, J. & Brent, M. *Access Denied: Disabled People's Experience of Social Exclusion*. Leonard Cheshire, 1998
5. Daone, L. & Scott, R. *Ready, Willing and Disabled*. Scope, 2003
6. Labour Market Trends – June 2003
7. Labour Force Survey 2002: Great Britain
8. Daone, L. & Scott, R. Op. cit.
9. Ibid.
10. Lamb, B. & Layzell, S. *Disabled in Britain: A World Apart.* Scope, 1994
11. Stewart, J. *In Good Company?* Scope, 1996
12. Morris, G. & Ford, J. Left out – disabled people's access to goods and services. Scope, 2000.
13. Lamb, B. & Layzell, S. *Disabled in Britain: behind closed doors.* Scope, 1995
14. *Eight hours a day and taken for granted?* The Princess Royal Trust for Carers, 1998
15. Lamb, B. & Layzell, S. Op.cit.
16. Ibid.

- The above information is from Scope's website which can be found at www.scope.org.uk

© Scope

Action needed to improve disabled people's lives

Information from the Prime Minister's Strategy Unit

Disabled people fare less well compared to non-disabled people and new action is needed to remove barriers and improve outcomes for disabled people, highlights an interim report released 16 June 2004 by the Prime Minister's Strategy Unit.

The Analytical Report 'Improving the Life Chances of Disabled People' has identified that around 10 million people are affected by disability including almost 20% of the UK working-age population, with trends suggesting this is on the increase.

Sponsor Minister, Maria Eagle, said: 'The Government is committed to improving the opportunities for disabled people and that is why the Strategy Unit has been commissioned to undertake this review.

'With such a large proportion of our population and workers affected by disability, it is vital that we identify major changes to reduce barriers that inhibit people from participating within our community.

'This work will promote a greater understanding of disability and provide practical solutions to ensure a more positive experience and understanding of disability in our society.

'I encourage all interested parties to respond to the issues raised in this Analytical Report, which will feed into the final recommendations.'

The report also identified the continuing situation where disabled people suffer adverse social outcomes, particularly at key transition points of their lives. This occurs when they move between full-time education and employment or between employment and economic inactivity.

Children with disabled parents and families with disabled children are also particularly affected, with 55% of families with disabled children living in or on the margins of poverty.

Also, while there are many successful government services and policies in place, these can be fragmented and their effectiveness can be low in some cases.

The overall aim of the project is to identify practical ways to remove barriers and improve outcomes for disabled people. Specifically it is exploring disabled people's 'life chances' and will make policy recommendations to government based around a comprehensive vision for disabled people. This will be achieved by:

Around 10 million people are affected by disability including almost 20% of the UK working-age population

- assessing the extent to which disabled people are suffering adverse economic and social outcomes in the UK;
- identifying why this is happening and what are its implications; and
- recommending what can be done to improve the situation.

The definition of a 'disabled' person includes a person with mental health conditions, long-term illness, learning difficulties and the effects brought on by old age.

Information and feedback from this Analytical Report will feed into the final report expected to be presented to the Government in autumn 2004.

- The above information is from the Prime Minister's Strategy Unit's website which can be found at www.strategy.gov.uk

Disability Living Allowance

Recipients of Disability Living Allowance (DLA): by main disabling condition, 2003[1,2]

Great Britain	Thousands
Arthritis	500.9
Other mental health causes[3]	334.3
Learning difficulties	239.2
Back ailments	216.5
Muscle/bone/joint disease	196.8
Heart disease	155.3
Stroke related	98.7
Chest disease	85.7
Blindness	60.4
Malignant disease	59.2
Epilepsy	57.1
Diabetes mellitus	46.8
Deafness	29.8
Parkinson's disease	13.6
Skin diseases	13.5
Renal disorders	11.5
AIDS	7.1
Other	342.6
All conditions	**2468.9**

1 At 28 February
2 Where more than one disability is present, only the main disabling condition is recorded.
3 Includes psychosis and dementia

Source: Department for Work and Pensions. Crown copyright.

Still itching for change

Information from RADAR

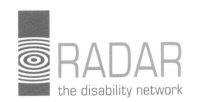

Our agenda-setting report 'Disability Discrimination: the Seven-Year Itch' (published in 2003) identified key areas for RADAR's campaigning work. Although progress has been made, we still have big ambitions in all those areas. From education to employment, housing to transport, we're still itching for change. These are some of the issues we'll be campaigning boldly on during 2004.

Education

The main aim of the Special Educational Needs and Disability Act 2001 was to increase inclusion in mainstream schools in the UK.

Fact: An increasing number of disabled children, their parents and other disabled people and disability organisations now support inclusive education.

RADAR is campaigning to highlight the many benefits of inclusive education for disabled children and for the education system. RADAR will launch a campaign, 'School Dinners', to bring together students, parents and teachers to report their experience of inclusive education to highlight best practice and recommend policy changes.

Employment

In October 2004 the provisions of the Disability Discrimination Act (DDA) will be extended to include employers with two or more employees. This will greatly increase the percentage of employers covered by the provisions of the DDA.

Fact: Many disabled people who would like to work are still unable to do so because of the inaccessibility of workplace buildings and the lack of awareness of many employers.

RADAR believes that disabled people should have the same access to employment as non-disabled people and will push for changes in workplace culture and more flexible working practices to enable disabled people to achieve this. RADAR will progress their 'First Hurdle' campaign to help recruitment agencies understand the needs and expectations of both disabled people and their forward-thinking business clients.

Transport

RADAR understands that the forthcoming Disability Bill should contain a number of important transport regulations. These include, for example, the setting of a date by which all rail vehicles should be accessible.

Fact: We are some way from an inclusive integrated transport system.

RADAR will campaign for an inclusive transport system, particularly for accessibility regulations for taxis, through our 'TAXI!' campaign. Similarly, RADAR will monitor the implementation and enforcement of a revised Blue Badge Parking Scheme and press for 2017 to be the end date by which all rail vehicles are accessible.

The built environment

The task of ensuring that buildings are built with at least a minimal level access is the responsibility of local authority Building Control Officers successfully enforcing Part M of the Building Regulations. In May 2004, the situation should improve when the regulations are extended to bring existing buildings undergoing alteration or change of use within the scope of Part M.

October 2004 will see the introduction of the final regulations under the DDA. Service providers will have to remove any physical barriers that prevent disabled people from accessing their services – or, alternatively, provide the same service by other means.

Fact: The current planning system plays scant regard to the needs of disabled people. On those occasions when developments meet or, still more rarely, go beyond, the requirements of Part M, it is frequently thanks to local access groups with RADAR's support rather than just council officials.

Together with other disability organisations and statutory bodies such as the Disability Rights Commission, RADAR will push on towards a planning system that will provide a genuinely accessible environment through, for example, the amendment of the current Planning and Compulsory Purchase Bill. RADAR's 'Access 04' campaign will gauge the readiness of local service providers for their forthcoming duties.

Housing

The Disability Discrimination Act 1995 and the extension of Part M of the Building Regulations in 1999 to cover new housing have helped to bring accessible housing to some disabled people.

Fact: For disabled people to live independently it is essential that they have a right to accessible and affordable housing.

RADAR will highlight the importance of Lifetime Homes standards – which guarantee full accessibility throughout one's life – as the minimum level of access provision in Part M of the Building Regulations. RADAR will urge that planning policy be used to ensure that it has 100% take-up by both the public and private sectors. As some wheelchair users are not able to use Lifetime Homes RADAR will also campaign for 10% of properties to be built to an agreed national wheel-chair standard.

Independent living

Government guidelines on charging and the increased availability of direct payments, whereby local authority money to meet the additional costs of disability is paid to the disabled person rather than to the service provider, have enabled some disabled people to live independently more successfully.

Fact: Although most disabled people now want and expect to live independently in their local communities, there are a host of problems with the current system. Some disabled people still cannot access direct payments and despite government guidelines, some disabled people on low incomes are still being overcharged for services.

RADAR will forge links with the National Centre for Independent Living to campaign for adequate support for disabled people to live independently and meet their personal and domestic needs as they require, for direct payments and against unfair charges.

Economic independence

In recent years, improved regulations, flexibility and awareness among benefits authorities and employers have enabled more disabled people to achieve economic independence.

Fact: Most disabled people in the UK face financial hardship through a combination of low benefits or low paid employment, as well as the extra cost incurred because of disability.

RADAR will continue to work with the Disability Alliance to campaign for Disability Living Allowance and other benefits to be increased to reflect the true costs of disability; for Winter Fuel Payments to be extended to severely disabled children and adults of working age; and for the government to take steps to ensure that there is a greater take-up of benefits by those who are entitled.

Politics and legislation

The UK's first-ever Disability

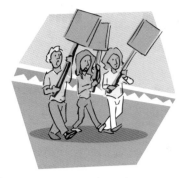

Discrimination legislation was enacted in 1995.

RADAR believes that the DDA 1995 was only a small step along the road to disabled people getting full civil rights. Over the coming months, alongside other disability organisations, RADAR will be working to ensure that the recently announced disability bill is not only robust but is as great a step as possible towards achieving full civil rights.

Information

The Disability Discrimination Act has helped open the door to information for some disabled people.

Fact: The door has been opened but not wide enough for all disabled people to go through it. Information is key in the knowledge economy and disabled people continue to have to put up with poor or inaccurate information which, despite the provisions of the DDA, is often available only in totally inaccessible formats.

RADAR will campaign for both a greater awareness of the needs of the end-user and for their experience to form the basis of information production.

Health

The NHS is becoming better at listening to disabled people and responding to their, sometimes, acute health problems.

Fact: Because the NHS remains largely focused on the treatment of acute health problems, it is less concerned with the ongoing health needs of the majority of disabled people.

RADAR will continue to campaign to make the NHS aware of the benefits of providing quality assistive technology to reduce the cost of disability both to the individual and the health service. RADAR is considering the development of best practice information to help disabled people use the NHS complaints procedures.

By becoming a member of RADAR you are supporting the campaign for social inclusion of disabled people. Today, not tomorrow.

■ The above information is from *Today, not tomorrow*, produced by RADAR. For more information visit their website at www.radar.org.uk

© RADAR

Economic activity

Economic activity status of working-age people:[1] by sex and whether disabled,[2] 2003[3]

United Kingdom	Men		Women		All	Percentages
	Disabled	Not disabled	Disabled	Not disabled	Disabled	Not disabled
Economically active						
In employment	51	86	46	75	49	81
Unemployed	5	4	3	3	4	4
All economically active	57	90	49	78	53	85
Economically inactive						
Wants a job	15	2	15	5	15	4
Does not want a job	28	7	36	17	32	12
All economically inactive	43	10	51	22	47	15

1 Males aged 16 to 64, females aged 16 to 59.
2 Current long-term health problem or disability.
3 At spring. Data are not seasonally adjusted and have not been adjusted to take account of the Census 2001 results. See Appendix, Part 4: LFS reweighting.

Source: Labour Force Survey, Office for National Statistics. Crown copyright.

Disability discrimination

Information from the Advisory, Conciliation and Arbitration Service

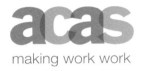

What is a disability?

For the purposes of the Disability Discrimination Act, disability is defined as a physical or mental impairment which has a substantial and long-term adverse effect on a person's ability to carry out their normal day-to-day activities.

What does the Disability Discrimination Act do?

The Disability Discrimination Act 1995 makes it unlawful for employers to discriminate against current or prospective workers who have a disability or who have had a disability in the past. This applies only to employers with 15 or more employees. The employer also has a duty under the Disability Discrimination Act to make reasonable adjustments to either the workplace, workstation or working environment to help the disabled person cope with their disability. However, businesses employing fewer than 15 people may wish, as good practice, to ensure that their present employment arrangements do not discriminate against people with disabilities.

When does discrimination occur?

When an employer treats a person with a disability less favourably than he treats other people and this treatment cannot be justified. Discrimination also occurs if an employer fails to comply with a duty to make a reasonable adjustment in relation to the disabled person and the failure to do so cannot be justified.

What is a 'reasonable adjustment'?

A reasonable adjustment is any step(s) that it is reasonable to have to take in all the circumstances. These adjustments should ensure that employment arrangements or premises do not put a disabled person at a disadvantage in comparison to a non-disabled person. An employment tribunal would look at all the circumstances of the case before making a decision as to what constituted reasonable adjustments. For example, things that may have a bearing would be the financial cost of the adjustment, the resources of the employer, practicability of the adjustment and the availability to the employer of financial or other assistance to help make an adjustment.

Can people make claims to employment tribunals under the Act?

People who have a disability as defined, who believe they have been the subject of discrimination in employment matters or consider a reasonable adjustment has not been made, may complain to an employment tribunal. There are no length of service or age requirements and the individual does not have to have left employment. The claim must be made within three months from when the discrimination took place.

Where can you get more information?

The Disability Rights Commission can provide more detailed guidance. Their helpline is 0845 7622 633 or textphone 0845 7622 644. The website is www.drc-gb.org Particularly useful leaflets are:
DL170 *Disability Discrimination Act 1995: What Employers need to know*
DLE 7 *Employing Disabled People: A good practice guide for managers and employers*
DLE 9 *Disability Discrimination Act 1995: An Introduction for small and medium sized businesses – Rights of Access to goods, facilities, services and premises*

Equality Direct provides free advice for businesses on equality issues. Trained advisers can be contacted on 08456 00 34 44.

■ The above information is from the Advisory, Conciliation and Arbitration Service's website which can be found at www.acas.org.uk
© *Advisory, Conciliation and Arbitration Service (Acas)*

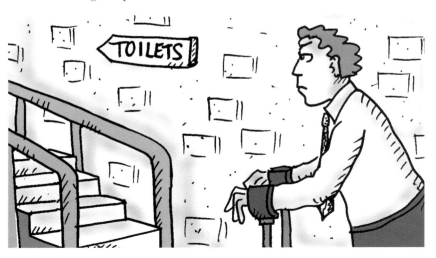

Open 4 all

2004 and disabled people

From 1 October 2004, disabled people have new rights of access of goods, services, facilities and premises. Here are answers to some key questions about your rights:

How does the Act define 'disabled people'?

You are protected from discrimination under the DDA if you have a physical or mental impairment that affects your ability to carry out normal day-to-day activities. That effect must be:

- Substantial (that is, more than minor or trivial) and;
- Adverse and;
- Long term (lasting or likely to last for at least a year). This means that not only do people with mobility impairments have rights but also disabled people with sensory impairments, learning difficulties or mental health issues, as well as many other disabled people.

What are 'goods and services' under the Act?

Most services are covered by the DDA. Anyone who provides a service to the public or a section of the public is a service provider. There are a few exceptions: private clubs

> Disability Rights Commission

that have a meaningful selection process for members, transport (but only the transport vehicle, not everything else connected with it such as stations, airports and booking facilities) and education (but there will be new DDA duties from September 2002). Not all manufactured goods are covered. The maker of a bathroom suite does not have to make the bath accessible for you but the shop selling it has to make sure that it is not unreasonably difficult to use its services. It doesn't matter whether or not you pay for the service; it's providing the service that matters. So disabled people have rights to all kinds of services. That includes going to a restaurant, shopping for clothes or food, using the local library, going to church or visiting your solicitor or doctor. All of these people provide services and are covered by Part III of the DDA.

The 2004 duties say that service providers should make reasonable adjustments to physical features but what is a physical feature?

Here is a long but not exhaustive list: steps, stairways, kerbs, exterior surfaces and paving, parking areas, building entrances and exits (including emergency escape routes), internal and external doors, gates, toilet and washing facilities, public facilities (such as telephones, counters or service desks), lighting and ventilation, lifts and escalators. It is important to realise that these features aren't just buildings or indoor facilities. They include seating in the street or a pub garden, stiles and paths in a country park, or fixed signs in a shop or leisure facility.

Do service providers only have to make changes when it's completely impossible for me to use their services?

No. They also have to make changes when it's unreasonably difficult. They should think about whether your time, inconvenience, effort, discomfort or loss of dignity in using the service would be considered unreasonable by other people if they had to endure similar difficulties.

Service providers are expected to make 'reasonable adjustments' to physical features but what is 'reasonable'? This isn't something we can give a straight answer to. The law uses this phrase to allow different solutions in different situations. However, the Code of Practice does say that what is reasonable may vary according to:

- The type of services being provided,
- The nature of the service provider and its size and resources,
- The effect of the disability on you.

These are some of the factors that service providers might have to take into account:

- Whether taking particular steps would overcome the difficulty that you face in accessing their service,
- How practicable it is to take the steps,

The Disability Discrimination Act

The Disability Discrimination Act (DDA) gives disabled people rights in the way they receive goods, services or facilities. Service providers already have to change the way they deliver their services if they are difficult for disabled people to use. Your rights to services have been introduced in three stages:

1. Since 2 December 1996 it has been against the law for service providers to treat you less favourably because of your disability.
2. Since 1 October 1999 service providers have had to make 'reasonable adjustments' for you, such as giving extra help or changing the way they provide their services.
3. From 1 October 2004 service providers may have to make other 'reasonable adjustments' to their premises so that there are no physical barriers stopping you from using or making it unreasonably difficult for you to use services.

The DRC have produced a new Code of Practice for service providers about the DDA. It will be taken into account by the courts where relevant and it guides disabled people and service providers on how reasonable adjustments should be made.

- The financial and other costs of this,
- How disruptive it would be,
- How much money and other resources they have available to spend on it,
- How much they have already spent,
- What financial help is available to them.

So you need to think about these factors when looking at whether the service is reasonable.

If a service provider does nothing until you are unable to use their services they could well be in breach of the law.

Is it OK for service providers to wait until I cannot use their services before making changes?

No. Their duties are anticipatory and continuing. In other words, service providers should be thinking ahead and continually looking at the way they provide services, their premises and the physical features and considering improvements for disabled people.

Can service providers just make changes for people with particular disabilities?

No. Service providers should not focus on stereotypes but should consider the full range of access needs of disabled people and the ways in which their services may be difficult to use. The DRC recommends that service providers have an access audit done. It is important to take into account the needs of a range of disabled people and not rely on stereotypes. As a disabled person you may want to become involved in this through your local access group or organisation.

Is it OK for service providers not to start thinking about this until October 2004?

Although the duties on physical features don't come into force until October 2004 service providers should be considering changes before then. They have been given lots of time by the government to assess what needs to be done and then prepare. The courts may well take into account what preparations, planning and changes service providers made in the period before October 2004 when considering whether they have met their legal duties.

How should a service provider deal with a physical feature that is making it difficult for me to use a service?

Once a service provider has identified the physical features that may make it difficult for you to use their service then the law gives them a choice. They can remove that feature, alter it, find a way of avoiding it or provide the service another way. The DRC strongly recommends that service providers first consider removing the physical feature or altering it. This is often the safest option because it is more likely to make the service accessible, meaning that you receive the services in the same way as other customers. This is called an 'inclusive' approach.

Where a service provider does decide to avoid a feature or provide the service another way, then the service must not be unreasonably difficult for you to use.

- The above information is from the Disability Rights Commission's website which can be found at www.drc-gb.org Alternatively see their address details on page 41.

© *Disability Rights Commission (DRC)*

Disability in the UK

Some facts and figures

- there are approximately 10 million disabled adults in Great Britain covered by the Disability Discrimination Act, which represents around 18 per cent of the population
- over 6.9 million disabled people are of working age which represents 20 per cent of the working population
- however, only 48 per cent of disabled people of working age are in employment compared to 82 per cent of non-disabled people of working age
- disabled people are nearly five times as likely as non-disabled people to be out of work and claiming benefits. Of the 2.9 million disabled people on state benefits and not in work over a million would like to work
- fewer than 8 per cent of disabled people use wheelchairs
- in 2004 40% of the English population are over 45, the age at which the incidence of disability begins to increase
- one in every four customers either has a disability or has a close relative or friend who is disabled
- the estimated annual purchasing power of people with disabilities is £40-£50 billion.

Statistics from the ONS, NCSR, RADAR, EFD

- The above information is from the Employers' Forum on Disability's website which can be found at www.employers-forum.co.uk

© *Employers' Forum on Disability 2004*

How to get in on the Disability Act

Is it just more red tape or could new laws championing disabled people actually profit small companies? Richard Tyler investigates

The Disability Discrimination Act extends to firms employing fewer than 15 staff in October and requires all businesses to provide equal physical access to their products and services or face the threat of prosecution.

This latest piece of regulation, which has been introduced in stages since 1996, appears to be full of pitfalls for small firms. In particular, the key test of whether an employer has acted 'reasonably' to provide his services or products to a disabled person will have to be tested in court in each disputed case.

The changes mean that as of October 1, firms with fewer than 15 staff have to treat job applications from disabled people on an equal basis to able-bodied candidates. They will also have to make all 'reasonable' alterations to the workplace for the benefit of existing disabled members of staff.

This includes physical access and suitable work practices such as the use of larger type in memos for partially sighted workers or vibrating fire alarms to aid deaf workers.

Firms have been banned since 1999 from enforcing policies that prevent disabled customers using their services. So a shop that refuses to admit dogs has to make an exception for a guide dog. But employers will now have to deal with all physical obstacles to service provision, such as steps, narrow corridors or a lack of lifts. A firm must either remove the obstacle, alter it or provide the service in another way, such as over the internet.

Business lobby groups acknowledge the point made by the government-funded Disability Rights Commission that many small firms are turning their back on the £50 billion annual spending power of the 8.6m seriously disabled people

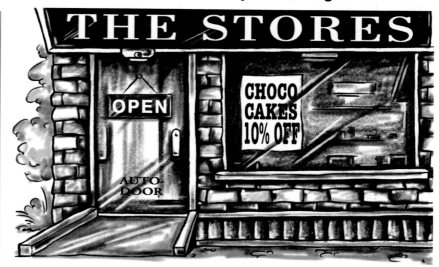

in the UK. But the Federation of Small Businesses also insists the Government has not fully appreciated the 'genuine cost implications' of making physical changes to service delivery.

It has lobbied the Treasury to allow firms to write off the cost of the investment against their taxable income, but to no avail. 'We are disappointed because it is a tried and tested route and it would fit in with the Government's agenda,' said spokesman David Bishop.

The Department for Work and Pensions says the new rules 'should not come as a surprise' to firms. 'The DDA is not about putting people out of business,' a spokesman said. But despite the lengthy run-up to implementation and significant sums of public money spent to spread the message, uncertainty over how to interpret the Act remains.

Battle Chamber of Commerce secretary Colin Smith said members attended a seminar last year organised by Hastings Enterprise that advised firms operating in conservation areas on how to approach the regulation. 'We were told that as long as you make some effort to meet the needs of the disabled then you have met the requirements of the Act,' said Mr Smith. 'It has been recognised that in towns like Battle and Rye the same rules cannot apply. It's impossible.'

Mr Smith said shops in listed buildings that could not improve access for wheelchairs could provide an alternative, such as installing a bell at the entrance so staff could serve the customer in the street. But Helen Kane, of commercial property expert Donaldsons, said the Act did not make any 'exemptions' for listed buildings. 'You still have to go through with the audit,' she said.

The access audit is one way employers can safeguard against future claims, though the DRC warns that an audit report does not constitute a watertight defence. Businesses are also advised to buy a copy of the DRC's code of practice, adherence to which will be seen as a plus in court.

The DRC has set up a national register of auditors who will, for a fee, establish whether a business measures up. Its own literature suggests the smallest firms need not go to the expense of an audit but should instead read the guides on its website.

To illustrate a suitable approach, the DRC cites the case of a small beauty salon that has a step at its entrance and limited space inside. The owners have already installed handrails to help customers up the step, and lowered the door bell. They then draw up a list of changes and remove the large mirrors in the foyer which the DRC says could confuse visually impaired people.

When the firm next redecorates it improves the colour contrast in the salon and changes the door handles, signs and toilet facilities.

Many small firms already recognise the business case for employing disabled staff and catering for their needs as customers. Shropshire-based Norman and Teresa Pearce altered their 16th-century public house, the Sun Inn, to cater for disabled and elderly patrons over eight years ago.

Mr Pearce widened the front door and made the pub's four levels accessible by ramps. He also pays attention to detail, such as using pint glasses with easy-to-hold handles. 'People are scared of [the legislation] but when I go into a pub or a shop I see that it can be completely wheelchair friendly for the cost of a bag of cement,' he said.

Firms have been banned since 1999 from enforcing policies that prevent disabled customers using their services

---

Mr Pearce said he would see changing a few steps into a ramp as 'reasonable' but thought 'it would probably not be reasonable' to expect a business to alter say 10 steps because, in the case of a pub, it would mean a significant loss of table space.

He said it was logical to make his business as customer-friendly as possible. 'We get a lot of elderly people coming to Shropshire on holiday. If you have a family of four and you can't let the wheelchair through, you lose the family,' he said.

Useful links

- Access to Work – advice and grants for employers hiring disabled staff. Go to the 'employers' section of www.jobcentreplus.gov.uk
- DisabledGo – local guides to firms supplying goods and services that have been made accessible to disabled people: www.disabledgo.info
- Typetalk/TextDirect – a service for deaf people to access goods and services over the telephone. Firms can contact deaf customers using the BT-operated service by adding the prefix 18002 before their number. Typetalk offers a free training service for firms. Call 0800 7311 888.
- Employers' Forum on Disability: www.employers-forum.co.uk

Single body will cover all acts of discrimination

By Sarah Womack, Social Affairs Correspondent

Ministers announced controversial plans 30 October 2003 for a single equality and human rights body to tackle all forms of discrimination.

The Commission for Equality and Human Rights will replace separate organisations currently dealing with discrimination against women, ethnic minorities and the disabled.

The Government says it will remove the need for the Commission for Racial Equality, the Disability Rights Commission and the Equal Opportunities Commission when it is formally launched in 2006.

The new commission will also deal with age, religious and sexual orientation discrimination, which are set to be covered by new European directives in the next few years.

It is the prospect of new directives that has spurred ministers to act.

Supporters of the Government's plans say they will help people who face discrimination for more than one reason.

But the move has upset some disability rights and sexual equality campaigners who fear the expertise of an individual body will be lost.

Bert Massie, chairman of the Disability Rights Commission, said a single 'gateway' could not cope with the vast range of different issues.

The commission had wanted a single group with an umbrella body sharing resources for staff recruitment, finance and a helpline.

Its proposed body was different from the Government's in that it would also include specialist units for each type of discrimination.

The Equal Opportunities Commission said a single body that was not backed up by stronger laws on sexual equality would send a message to women that the Government did not regard sex equality as a priority.

However, Help the Aged said the new body would ensure greater consistency and be more powerful in helping to change public attitudes. The Commission for Racial Equality declined to comment on the Government's proposals until after they were published.

Making new laws to protect disabled people

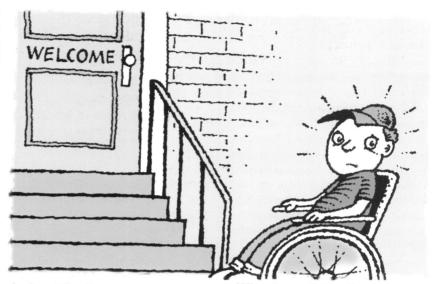

The Government wants to make some new laws

There are already laws to make sure that disabled people are treated fairly. These laws help when a disabled person can't use a service like a pub or a bank just because they are disabled.

The Government wants to make new laws for disabled people. These new laws will make sure that disabled people are treated fairly in a lot more ways.

What are the new laws the Government wants to make?

The Government wants to make sure that people who provide transport to the public treat disabled people fairly. This will mean that disabled people cannot be stopped from travelling on things like trains, buses, coaches and aeroplanes just because they are disabled.

The law already makes sure that people who provide public services, like Councils or the police, or the National Health Service, must treat disabled people fairly in most things they do. The Government wants to make this law even better so that public bodies treat disabled people fairly all the time. And it wants the people who run these services to make sure that they think about disabled people when they try to make the services work better.

The law already makes sure that landlords must treat disabled people fairly when renting houses or flats to them. The Government wants to make this law even better so that landlords must look at how they rent property to disabled people. For example, a landlord might have to read out any letter he writes about the rent.

The Government also wants to make sure that the law looks after more disabled people. At the moment, some people who have HIV, cancer or Multiple Sclerosis don't always count as disabled under the law. The Government wants to change this so that more of those people are counted as disabled by the law and treated fairly.

The Government wants to make sure that clubs, such as a sports club with 25 or more members, treat disabled people fairly. This will mean that a club cannot refuse to let a person be a member just because they have a disability, unless they have a very good reason.

The Government wants to make new laws for disabled people. These new laws will make sure that disabled people are treated fairly in a lot more ways

---

The Government also wants to make sure that local Councils treat elected local Councillors who are disabled fairly. This will help disabled Councillors carry out their duties properly.

The new laws will also make some other changes to help disabled people.

Why doesn't the Government just make these laws?

The Government wants to test the laws first to make sure that they will work properly. They have written down the laws in what is called a draft Bill.

This will give the people in Parliament a chance to look at the laws and ask some questions about them.

If you want to see the draft Bill, its full name is the Draft Disability Discrimination Bill. You can get a copy from: The Stationery Office (TSO) 0870 600 5522 www.tso.co.uk

Getting help

Disabled people who want to know more about how the law already helps them can get advice from the Disability Rights Commission: 08457 622 633 www.drc-gb.org

Want to know more about these new laws?

If you would like to know more about how these new laws might work, please contact:

Department for Work and Pensions, Disability Unit, 6th Floor, The Adelphi, 1-11 John Adam Street, London WC2N 6HT or phone on: 020 7962 8650

© Crown copyright

Disabled children left out in the cold again?

The Children Bill is currently going through Parliament. But unless the concerns of disability groups are addressed, there is a real danger disabled children will miss out again

By Angus Baldwin, Parliamentary Officer

When Victoria Climbié died aged eight years old in February 2000 she had 128 separate injuries to her body inflicted by her guardians. The young girl was known to four social services departments, three housing departments, two specialist child protection teams of the Metropolitan Police, two hospitals and a families centre managed by the NSPCC and yet she still suffered unimaginable cruelty over many months before she was finally murdered.

It was clear that something had gone horribly wrong with a system which had been designed specifically to prevent such tragedies. The outcry led to much soul-searching amongst politicians and child care professionals, an official inquiry, a Green Paper *Every Child Matters* and now a new Children Bill which was introduced into the House of Lords at the end of March.

The Bill is an attempt not only to try and make sure that another child does not suffer the same awful fate as Victoria but also to try and ensure that every child has the best life chances possible. So the Bill establishes new 'Local Safeguarding Children Boards' for every local authority to protect vulnerable children. But it also creates a new UK Children's Commissioner to promote the views and interests of children, and sets out five areas where children's services must improve young people's 'well-being', namely physical and mental health, protection from harm and neglect, education and training, the contribution made by them to society and their social and economic well-being. This new vision – of both protection and improving life chances – is one we are passionately in favour of. But we are worried that unless disabled children are placed firmly at the heart of this Bill, they will lose out as children's services focus their efforts on non-disabled children – as happens currently.

We helped produce the recent National Working Group on Child Protection and Disability report *It doesn't happen to disabled children* which highlighted that disabled children are over three times more likely to be abused or neglected than non-disabled children. That's why Mencap is pressing the Government for the new Children's Boards to have at least one expert on disabled children on them.

We also want disabled children not only to be involved in the appointment of the new Commissioner but also to be central to everything that he or she then does. For this to happen, the Commissioner will need to proactively seek the views of all groups of children including children with more severe or profound learning disabilities. And all consultation processes, complaints procedures and key documents must be fully accessible.

Lord Rix and others will be pressing our case in the House of Lords as the Bill goes through Parliament during May and June. What seems likely is that without special treatment disabled children will get left behind again and the gap between their life chances and those of non-disabled children will grow ever wider. And if that happens, the Children Bill will have singularly failed and a once-in-a-generation opportunity will have been missed.

Key points

- The Government has published the Children Bill which is now going through Parliament.
- Mencap is concerned that the Bill does not contain enough about disabled children.
- Unless disabled children's needs are placed firmly in the Bill, the Government will once again fail to treat disabled children equally.
- The Children Bill is at: www.publications.parliament.uk/pa/pabills.htm

■ The above information is from *Viewpoint* May/Jun 2004, the magazine produced by Mencap. For more information visit their website: www.mencap.org.uk

© Mencap

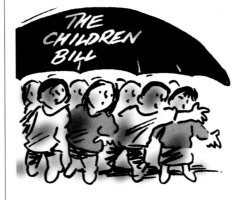

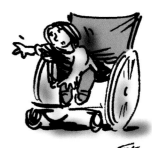

To be or not to be honest?

Graduates with disabilities fear discrimination at job interviews

By Kate Crockett

To disclose or not to disclose: that is the question facing every disabled candidate tackling the graduate recruitment process. 'I don't like to disclose my disability,' says Paul, an economic history graduate from London School of Economics, who is partially sighted.

'I don't trust people, to be honest. I feel it tarnishes their views of me. I've seen it before outside the workplace so why should it be any different within the workplace?'

Paul's experience isn't unique. 'The reasons people don't want to disclose are because they don't want to be discriminated against, they don't want to be different, or, quite often, because they feel it is nobody else's business,' says Tab Ahmad, graduate development manager for national charity Employment Opportunities, which advises both candidates and employers, such as the Civil Service, MI5, Procter and Gamble, Barclays and HSBC, on disability and employment issues.

However, as Paul has found, it isn't always possible to avoid disclosing a disability on a carefully worded application form, without lying. This is because disclosure is also a big issue for recruiters. Employers ask 'the disability question' to make any necessary adjustments to the subsequent recruitment processes and, if the candidate is successful, in the workplace. They also monitor applications from disabled candidates, as they do from ethnic minorities, for equal opportunities reasons.

However, while respectable employers will use this information appropriately, applicants can never know for certain if disclosure will have a negative impact on their chances. 'There is a need to develop more trust between applicants and recruiters so that people can declare disabilities and not expect that this will put them in the "no" pile,' explains Barbara Waters, chief executive of Skill, the national bureau for students with disabilities. 'Recruiters need to show that they have taken on-board the "ability is what counts" message.'

And this is where good-practice employers are focusing their energy – building a dialogue with candidates to address concerns and to demonstrate the practical steps they are taking to remove any existing physical or organisational barriers to work. Some organisations are doing so by achieving the 'two ticks' kitemark, which indicates that they are positive about employing staff with disabilities, while others are involved in graduate-specific initiatives.

> '*There is a need to develop more trust between applicants and recruiters so that people can declare disabilities and not expect that this will put them in the "no" pile*'

The Open University, Bupa, Ford, Corus, Kodak, B&Q and the Department for Education and Skills are among the diverse range of partner organisations in the Fast-Track scheme, run by the charity

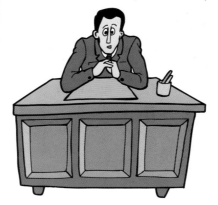

Scope, which offers work placements to disabled graduates. Candidates are recruited by Scope to undertake two six-month paid placements in different organisations, gaining valuable work experience and training.

The placements do not guarantee a job on completion, but up to 70% of Fast-Track graduates gain full-time employment with a host employer.

Amelia Jarman, a 25-year-old chemistry graduate from Edinburgh university, is currently on her first six-month Fast-Track placement at B&Q's headquarters in Southampton. Amelia, who has epilepsy and dyslexia, graduated in 2000 but since then had been working in a pub, having had only one other unsuitable job offer. 'I was offered very few interviews and, when I was, the jobs didn't fully utilise my skills and knowledge,' Amelia explains.

Now, she is using her subject expertise in B&Q's social responsibility department identifying chemicals in products and recommending how their environmental impact can be reduced. 'Many companies are not confident about handling disability, and lack of experience has a lot to do with this,' she continues. 'I hope B&Q's involvement will encourage more companies to feel positive about employing disabled people.'

B&Q's policy of embracing diversity, through initiatives such as Fast-Track scheme and targeting older workers, is a proven success and has strengthened the business case for diversity strategies. Gradually, an increasing number of organisations in sectors not traditionally considered diverse are recognising the benefits of recruiting from a wider talent pool.

The Capital Chances event, which is run by graduate-specialist publisher GTI, has, in the past, given the investment banking sector a chance to promote itself to female and ethnic minority applicants. This month, Capital Chances is targeting disabled students with a one-day event involving business games and simulations mirroring the work of corporate financiers, and providing the opportunity for candidates to find out more about employment opportunities at Goldman Sachs, HSBC, JP Morgan, Merrill Lynch, Morgan Stanley and UBS.

'The reason they are doing this is because they realise that they haven't actually been getting to people that they might need and that the best person for the job isn't necessarily coming forward via the process they were using before,' says Barbara Waters of Skill, which is supporting the event.

Stephanie Allwood, diversity recruiter at UBS, continues: 'We see the Capital Chances event as very much a two-way communication vehicle, not only as an opportunity for the students to find out about banking, but also for us to find out what perceptions the students may have of our industry, work environment and selection process.'

'It gives disabled students the chance to explore career opportunities and allows better understanding between investment banks and disabled graduates to make a better working environment for all,' agrees Matthew Johnson, a senior associate in IT at Morgan Stanley, and graduate of Oxford Brookes.

Matthew, who is hearing impaired, advises potential candidates: 'Investment banks tend to recruit people who work well in a team and have the ability to meet tight deadlines. To succeed you should be honest with yourself and that means being open about your disability with your colleagues. You must have a "can do" attitude.'

That 'can do' attitude is what all graduates strive to demonstrate to employers, but the challenge remains to convince employers that, for disabled recruits, 'can't do one thing' doesn't mean 'can't do anything'.

Keziah Halliday, a European studies finalist at University College London, says: 'I think the main barrier to employing people with disabilities isn't prejudice – although there is still a lot of that around. It is actually ignorance and a lack of willing to make changes to make it possible to employ people with disabilities.'

Keziah, who is 23 and has a congenital absence of the left hand and forearm, continues: 'I don't really require any modifications or adaptations, so employing me is, to all intents and purposes, the same as employing an able-bodied person. Even so, I fall into the disabled category with all the highs and lows that that entails.'

But, for Keziah now, it's a high – she's made it through the first stages of the Civil Service Fast Stream selection process and is pinning her hopes on success at its April selection board.

■ This article first appeared in the *Guardian*, 8 March 2003.

© Kate Crockett

Disabled people as workers

Information from the Employers' Forum on Disability

■ there are 6.9 million disabled people of working age in the UK, 19 per cent of the working population (Labour Force Survey summer 2003).

■ disabled people in employment tend to work in a similar range of jobs to non-disabled people and can offer employers exactly the same range of skills and talents as anyone else. They often have additional problem-solving skills developed from managing their everyday life. Yet unemployment rates among people with disabilities are around twice those for non-disabled people.

■ disabled people tend to be more loyal than many other workers and have a tendency to remain with employers for longer periods.

■ disabled people have fewer days off sick and fewer days' absence for reasons other than illness compared to non-disabled workers, their productivity rates are on a par with other workers and they have better than average safety records.

■ disabled employees have the same aspirations and ambitions as anyone else in the workforce. They want jobs which are challenging and rewarding and are just as likely to want opportunities for career development and promotion.

■ 7 out of 10 economically active disabled people of working age will have become disabled during their working life. Losing the services of an employee who becomes disabled deprives organisations of a considerable asset and investment in terms of their skills and experience. It can also be very expensive. One large employer found that the average cost of retiring an employee on medical grounds was £40,000.

■ 1 out of every 4 customers is disabled or has a disabled person in their immediate circle. The value of the disability market in the UK is estimated to be £40 billion per annum. Organisations that employ disabled people are better able to anticipate and respond to the needs of disabled customers. They have in their disabled employees an inbuilt source of information and advice about their potential customers on which they can draw in developing their marketing strategies.

■ The above information is from the Employers' Forum on Disability's website which can be found at www.employers-forum.co.uk

© *Employers' Forum on Disability* 2004

Disability on TV

Six disabled teenagers have joined forces with the national children's charity Whizz-Kidz to host a conference about disability on TV. The conference, which was held in Birmingham on 21 November 2003, was unique in that it was organised by young people, for young people to challenge the current lack of representation of disabled people in mainstream television.

The young organisers, all of whom are wheelchair users themselves, decided to host the event after receiving the results of 'Disability on the Box' survey which they carried out in the Midlands with help from Whizz-Kidz. The survey showed that 70% of young people, both able-bodied and disabled, feel that attitudes towards disabled people would improve if there were more positive representations of them on television.

These conclusions mirror those obtained by the key players broadcast industry itself in a recent survey entitled 'Disabling Prejudice'. Both reports concur that young disabled people feel there should be more disabled people in mainstream television playing 'normal' roles that don't focus on their disability

The 'Disability on the Box' conference gave both disabled and able-bodied teenagers the unique chance to ask industry insiders about their current disability policies and make suggestions on how representation can be improved. As one of the problems highlighted by TV professionals is the lack of choice of disabled actors/presenters available, the participants also had the opportunity to join one of three interactive workshops in scriptwriting, advertising and acting/presenting. The idea of these workshops is to give a taster of what it is like to work in TV and the chance to develop potential storylines, which can be sent on to commissioning editors.

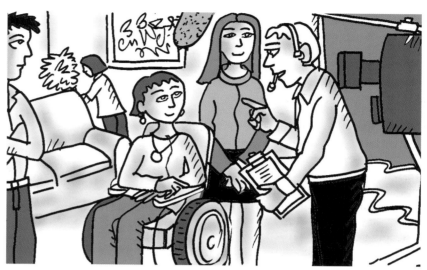

The event attracted a number of high-profile television names keen to give their advice and listen to the young people's opinions. These include: Steven Andrew, Controller of CiTV; Sue Caro, Senior Diversity Manager at the BBC; Richard Zajdlic, a script-writer for popular programmes such as *EastEnders* and *This Life*; comedian and actress Francesca Martinez, and Kim Tserkeize, star of children's BBC programme *Balamory*.

John Clarke, 15, one of the young organisers, says: 'Young disabled people don't often get the chance to talk with those who have the power to change things. We hope this conference will make a difference, not only by giving some good ideas to those in the television industry about how to include more disabled people in programmes, but also by encouraging more young disabled people apply for jobs in television so that they can help make a positive and active contribution.'

Julie Fernandez, star of TV's *The Office* and a supporter of Whizz-Kidz, adds: 'The television industry is committed to making more opportunities available for disabled people through the Broadcasting and Creative Industries Disability Network, but there is still a long way to go before there is regular representation of disabled people in mainstream television. There are still very limited opportunities available to disabled people wanting to work in television and to make matters worse disabled teenagers often have no access to advice on working in television or the opportunities that are available to them. I think this conference is a great idea and hope that it gives inspiration to young people.'

The conference is the third in a series of four regional events entitled 'Break Down Barriers' which are being funded by a Comic Relief grant. The grant was awarded to Whizz-Kidz to help enhance their consultation and networking with young people through the development of their 'Kidz Board' – a group of disabled teenagers who work as ambassadors and advisers to the charity.

Each conference is organised by a group of teenagers from the Kidz Board who are supported by a team at the charity's head office. A theme for each event is chosen because of its specific relevance to the lives of young disabled people and they aim to find ways to break down barriers to disabled people. Later in the year regional reports from each of the conferences will be combined into an overall national report, providing a definitive picture of young peoples' views on issues surrounding independent mobility within the UK.

Notes

- 200 teenagers were interviewed for the young people's survey, with a 60/40 split between disabled and able bodied, male and female.
- Seven out of ten respondents believe that able-bodied people's attitudes towards disabled people would improve if they regularly saw disabled people on TV.
- 60% of respondents think the best way of encouraging able-bodied people to see disabled people as 'normal' is to see them in main-

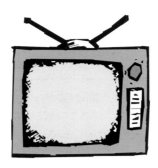

stream TV programmes where there is no focus on their disability.
- For two-thirds of young disabled people seeing disabled role models on TV has a positive effect inspiring them and making them hopeful that negative attitudes towards disabled people will change.

- Eight out of ten people could not recall any TV advertisements that featured disabled people and three-quarters think advertisers leave disabled people out of appearing in advertisements.
- Over half of young disabled respondents have been treated badly because of their disability. The culprits are most likely to be other young people or adults the respondents do not know.

■ The above information is from Whizz-Kidz's website which can be found at www.whizz-kidz.org.uk Visit the web site for a more detailed and informative report of this topic.
© 2004 Whizz-Kidz

Disablism

British public to test their attitudes towards disabled people

Scope has surveyed the British public to test their attitudes towards disabled people. Despite the achievements of Home Secretary David Blunkett, Professor Stephen Hawking and sportsperson Tanni Grey-Thompson, 36 per cent of those questioned in a YouGov survey could not name one single famous disabled person.

Two-thirds of those questioned believe it is acceptable for a non-disabled person to play the part of a disabled person in drama or film, despite it being generally considered highly offensive for a white actor to play the part of a black person today.

Scope argues that it is time to challenge this level of ignorance and prejudice and is calling for equality for disabled people who, at 10 million people, make up one of the largest minority groups still discriminated against in the UK today. As part of its drive to counter this, the charity launched a national advertising campaign, featuring disabled people telling their own stories and simply asking to be treated like other people.

The YouGov survey was carried out as part of Scope's Time to Get Equal campaign, which has the backing of Nelson Mandela, Prime Minister Tony Blair, the Home Secretary David Blunkett, Scope Patron Cherie Booth QC, former US President Bill Clinton and all the main political parties. Scope is calling for an end to disablism – discrimination against disabled people.

Some results were more positive: 87 per cent of people questioned by YouGov said that disabled people should have equal rights with non-disabled people and 40 per cent felt there aren't enough disabled people on television. However, when asked what they might do themselves to tackle the issue, responses were disappointing: 60 per cent were opposed to paying an extra supplement on council tax to ensure all public transport was accessible to disabled people. Scope has found that over 50 per cent of disabled people still face difficulties using public transport, keeping them excluded from society.

Tony Manwaring, chief executive of Scope, said:

'We are deeply concerned about the level of prejudice revealed by this report. The non-disabled public claims to believe in equality for disabled people, but once you look under the surface prevailing attitudes are shockingly outdated. The fact that so few people can actually name a famous disabled person demonstrates just how little value is placed on disabled people. Scope is working with disabled and non-disabled people to increase understanding with the aim of bringing about fundamental change at all levels of society.'

Scope is working with both non-disabled and disabled people to find ways of overcoming these barriers. To be part of the campaign to change people's attitudes and work towards a more inclusive and equal society, visit the Time to Get Equal website at: www.timetogetequal.org.uk

Members of the public can sign Scope's pledge to support disabled people achieving equality by texting: 'equality pledge' and your name to 60003 or call us on: 0845 355 0700 to request a pledge card. Alternatively they can visit one of Scope's 300 shops across England and Wales and request a pledge card.

■ The above information is from Scope's website which can be found at www.scope.org.uk
© Scope

Serious about laughter

Laughter is a release of tension. All of us tend to laugh most at things when we have some kind of deep-rooted anxiety about them. It's a great way to defuse serious issues. A real ice breaker

And there's nothing icy about Julie Fernandez. Familiar to comedy fans as Brenda in *The Office*, Julie has brittle bone disease, a condition which has meant that she has undergone more than seventy operations and gets around in a wheelchair. She bubbles with warmth, and is committed to the view that comedy can break down barriers.

She agrees that television in the UK has come a long way since *Crossroads*, when 'Sandy Richardson' climbed nimbly into his wheelchair to depict a supposedly positive image of disability, but adds that British casting directors are still wary of using truly disabled actors, recounting tales of parts not offered because the public are still frightened of their own insecurities about disability. It would be thought ridiculous now for white actors to put on make-up to play black parts, but there's no such attitude yet about portrayals of disabled people. So there is clearly still plenty of tension to be relieved.

Julie was born in London thirty years ago, but was soon on the move, living in South Africa, Germany and Spain before returning to England and attending a day school for disabled children in Essex. At the age of twelve she went to Treloar School where she was a member of the first class of disabled students to take GCSE Drama.

Julie's mother comes from Austria, and she was eager to study German at university at the completion of her sixth-form years, however it was almost impossible to find any university able to offer the course she wanted because of a widespread lack of access for students in wheelchairs.

> *It would be thought ridiculous now for white actors to put on make-up to play black parts, but there's no such attitude yet about portrayals of disabled people*

Just as she was seeing her options diminish, the BBC approached Treloar School because they wanted to cast a young disabled girl for the role of Liz Lochhead in *Eldorado* – a soap set in Spain which has become as legendary in TV folklore as *Crossroads*. Julie found herself almost accidentally starting a career in which rejection is commonplace, and talent needs to be matched with resolution and perseverance.

Not only has she achieved success as an actress, but she is also extremely active in working to improve life for disabled people, both by taking the opportunities her celebrity status gives to appear in the media to talk and write about disability issues, and by setting up The Disability Foundation, based at the Royal National Orthopaedic Hospital, Stanmore, to provide low-cost complementary therapies for people with disabilities.

Working on *The Office* has reunited Julie with another Old Treloarian. Ash Atalla, the show's producer, is also a wheelchair user, and Julie is keen to see the strengths of disabled people used more widely across the media. She has recently formed her own independent production company in partnership with Mick Scarlet, the BBC's leatherclad wheelchair-propelled iconoclastic former children's presenter, and is planning to make programs the like of which have never been seen before, with her sights firmly set upon mainstream TV comedy.

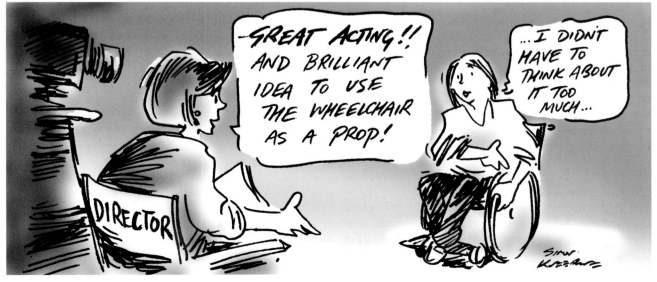

'The problem with disabled people in drama is that they're all either wicked villains like Captain Hook, or they're heroic stoic types,' says Julie, 'it's not very realistic. The problem is that most people feel more uncomfortable about disability, because there's a very real chance that it could happen to them. Any of us could give birth to a disabled child, all of us are going to grow old. It's not the same as colour, for example; there's no danger that, if you're black, you're going to wake up white one morning – unless of course you're Michael Jackson,' she giggles, 'but you could wake up disabled, and people don't want to be reminded of that.'

Julie feels that we've lost some of the open-mindedness that was more common in cultures that the modern world considers primitive and less 'civilised'.

'Before Christianity, religions used to value people who were different; in the old Celtic faiths they had power and were the strong ones because they had overcome their disabilities. Then Christianity came along and said "Oh, dear – you are sinners, confess and let us heal you".'

Julie believes that people fail to accept others' disabilities, even when they believe they accept the person themselves: 'It's wrong for disabled people to be considered as less worthy of treatment on the grounds that they will have less "Quality of Life Years" than somebody else – it's a dangerous step towards ideas of euthanasia being acceptable.'

'It's all a question of attitudes really. It's much better in the States. I was out there filming, and all the buses were accessible, with disabled people in the back – but the ADA came in and improved on that. They said "if everyone else gets on the front of the bus, then so should disabled people". And representation of disability in the media is much better. I'm in discussion at the moment about taking my acting career out to Hollywood, but that doesn't mean I'll be leaving the UK. My political career, fighting for the rights of disabled people in the UK, is just taking off, and there's still plenty of work to be done here.'

She has just co-written a comedy sketch show about disability for a mainstream audience, and is hopeful that, when aired, it will change attitudes in a similar way to the shift that has taken place as a result of *Goodness Gracious Me* and *The Kumars*.

'The problem is that most people feel more uncomfortable about disability, because there's a very real chance that it could happen to them. Any of us could give birth to a disabled child, all of us are going to grow old'

'As well as doing drama and more comedy in the future I want to move more into producing and writing. I find it equally exciting and important to be behind the camera as it is to be in front of it. I'm more business orientated; I really enjoy starting businesses, getting balls rolling and moving things forward. I think the trick is to know what you're good at.'

It's not just improved representation of disabled people on-screen that Julie wants to see. She believes there is a tremendous waste of our own resources through lack of accessibility to opportunites in higher education and in work, and feels that, before seeing asylum seekers as a source of workers to fill jobs needed

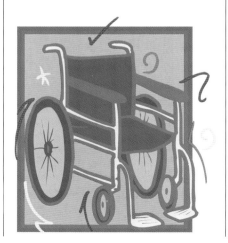

in our economy, we should be trying harder to fulfil the untapped potential of the many capable people with disabilities who are often frustrated by issues such as, for example, Access to Work benefits.

'I claim Access to Work benefits, but I have never had to deal with such an incompetent bunch of people in all my life!' says Julie. 'There are disabled people who can work, who want to work and who ought to take up these opportunities. Real integration means that disabled people need to be doing all sorts of jobs, and is not just about what we see on television screens. The requirements of the Disability Discrimination Act mean that disabled people now have the power to take legal action when they don't have access to opportunities, and the government need to make sure that they provide the funds needed to make accessibility a practical reality. It will mean building alterations at Universities, at workplaces and so on, plus a benefit system that is professionally applied and effective.'

Julie Fernandez may be a star, but it doesn't mean she has her head in the clouds; her ambitions have a scope that go far deeper than the provision of a little light relief from people's discomfort about disability. She sees the media as only a small part of her future. As an actor, presenter, writer, producer, journalist and prime mover of the Disability Foundation she already makes quite an impact, but there's clearly a lot more still to come.

'I deal with a lot of business people because of all the different things that I do, and I go to meetings. I know it "fazes" a lot of people; you know – the door opens and in comes a wheelchair user, four foot five, a young blonde woman – and I can see it in their eyes; "OK, so what are we going to get from this one?" but actually it gives me quite a voice!'

And it never harms to have a talented and energetic voice in our corner!

■ The above information is from Ability Media Ltd whose website can be found at www.ukability.co.uk

© Ability Media Ltd

Public transport?

Despite the UK's Government manifesto commitment in 2001 to implement all the Disability Rights Taskforce's outstanding recommendations relating to transport, there is a continued failure to do. Today eight and a half million – or one in seven of the UK population – are still struggling to get on board

Viv Spanton, a Londoner, a campaigner and a wheelchair user, has given up trying to use public transport. She finds even though London is one of the richest capitals in the world, its transport system is woefully inadequate. The lack of lifts and ramps makes much of the London Underground inaccessible and the irregularity of bus services makes them just too unreliable. And what's worse for Viv, is the generally rude, unhelpful and patronising attitudes of transport workers. 'The generally poor standards of public transport and patronising attitudes of workers makes getting around London impossible,' says Viv. 'I've been lucky enough to travel around America and Canada and I can go anywhere and do anything without having to worry about how I'm going to get there. New York City has a wonderful bus system – all the buses have ramps and the attitude of the drivers is far better than here.'

What Viv found in New York is that bus drivers were glad to help, rather than annoyed that they have to help as in the UK. She explains: 'Recently I was in Brighton with my husband for his great-great-niece's wedding. We found that accessible taxis in the city were few and far between, so we waited for a bus to get us to the wedding. When the bus pulled up, the driver refused to get the ramp out, saying he couldn't leave his money unattended. My husband was forced to lift me, in my wheelchair, onto the bus. The driver was so rude. When we had to get off the bus, the driver finally decided to help by putting the ramp out.'

The restrictions of travelling by train have had another effect on her life. Viv has found the staff more helpful and the trains more accessible than other modes of transport. She has to sit in 'special, dedicated areas' that are not integrated into general seating arrangements. But because she has to book days in advance to inform the guard that assistance is needed, she is unable to be spontaneous.

Viv explains: 'When I travel on trains, I have to plan ahead. I can't just get on, I can't be spontaneous. This means I don't see my friends as much as I like, as they believe I can't join in with last minute plans to meet up and socialise.' This situation is distressing for Viv.

Viv uses the Leonard Cheshire Day Service, Randall Close, in south west London, and supports Leonard Cheshire's new campaign for a fully accessible transport system. She says: 'Central government must create a public awareness programme to change the attitudes of transport companies and workers. Disabled people won't become fully integrated into public life until there's a transport system that enables them to get there.'

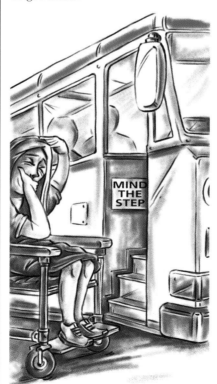

'The generally poor standards of public transport and patronising attitudes of workers makes getting around London impossible'

Mind the gap

In September 2003, Leonard Cheshire's Policy and Campaigns Team launched a report that outlined the social and emotional costs to disabled people of an inaccessible transport network. The report, *Mind The Gap*, reveals the disturbing truth that disabled people are having to miss medical appointments and social occasions with family and friends, as well as face unemployment, because the UK's current transport system is inaccessible to them.

Findings include:

- 23% of respondents that had sought employment during the last 12 months turned down a job offer because of inaccessible transport.
- 18% of respondents missed a medical appointment during the preceding two years because of difficulties caused by inaccessible transport.
- 25% of respondents do not see their family and friends as often as they'd like because they are restricted by inaccessible transport.

Leonard Cheshire's campaign is urging the Government to introduce measures that will deliver an accessible transport network as soon as possible. And put an end to one of the lasting barriers to disabled people's inclusion in society.

- The above article first appeared in Leonard Cheshire's magazine *Compass*. For a copy of *Mind The Gap* contact Leonard Cheshire. For their address details see page 41 or visit their website at www.leonard-cheshire.org

Statistics on learning disabilities

Some quick facts

What is meant by the term 'learning disabilities'?

The formal definition of 'learning disabilities' or 'intellectual disabilities' includes the presence of:

- a significant intellectual impairment and
- deficits in social functioning or adaptive behaviour
- which are present from childhood.

How many people in the UK have learning disabilities?

- There are no reliable official statistics concerning the number of people with learning disabilities in the UK.
- The estimated number of people with mild learning disabilities in the UK is 580,000-1,750,000. It is estimated 230,000-350,000 people have severe learning disabilities.
- The incidence of Down's syndrome is approximately 1 in 600.

Who has learning disabilities?

- Males are more likely than females to have both severe learning disabilities (average ratio 1.2 males: 1 female) and mild learning disabilities (average ratio 1.6 males: 1 female).
- Severe learning disabilities are more common among boys/men, young people and people from South Asian communities.
- Mild learning disabilities are more common among boys/men, young people, people who are poorer and people from adverse family backgrounds.

How many people have autistic spectrum disorders?

- Approximately 1 in 200 people have an autistic spectrum disorder.

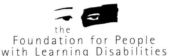

the
Foundation for People
with Learning Disabilities

- A greater number of boys than girls have autistic spectrum disorders. The male: female ratio is 3: 1 in children with autistic spectrum disorders and learning disabilities. This ratio is 6: 1 in children with autistic spectrum disorders and an IQ in the normal range.

What are the causes of learning disabilities?

- Biological, environmental and social factors are all involved in causing learning disabilities.
- Biological factors can be identified as causing severe learning disabilities in 4 out of 5 children and as causing mild learning disabilities in between 1 and 2 out of 5 children.

What are the health concerns of people with learning disabilities?

- 25-40 per cent of people with learning disabilities also have mental health problems.
- People with learning disabilities have a high level of unrecognised illness and have reduced access to generic preventative screening and health promotion procedures.

Are people with learning disabilities at risk of abuse?

- 23 per cent of adults with learning disabilities have experienced physical abuse.
- 47 per cent of adults with learning disabilities have experienced verbal abuse and bullying.

What is the cost of providing services to people with learning disabilities?

- Approximately £4.6 billion is spent a year to provide formal services for children and adults with learning disabilities in the UK.

- The above information is from the Foundation for People with Learning Disabilities' website: www.learningdisabilities.org.uk

© Foundation for People
with Learning Disabilities

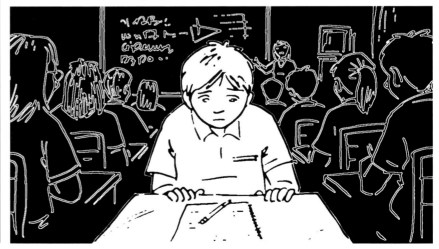

Understanding learning disabilities

Information from Mind (National Association for Mental Health)

This information is aimed at people who have a learning disability, their families and friends. It explains what it means, what some of the causes are, and what the effects may be. It also outlines some of the different kinds of support that are available to people who have these problems and their families, and how to access this.

What is a learning disability?

Someone who has a learning disability will have certain limitations on their ability to think (known as an impairment of intellectual ability). This limit might be hardly noticeable or very severe, and anywhere in between. In the past, there have been many other terms used, such as mental handicap and retardation. Those concerned find these labels offensive, and prefer to be described as having learning disabilities, or special needs.

These problems are often confused with mental illness, but they are quite different. A learning disability is a lifelong condition, which starts very early on. Unlike a mental illness, it doesn't cause an unstable personality, temporarily distort a person's view of the world, change dramatically or 'get better'. Although a learning disability can never go away, there's a great deal that can be done to support and enable people to lead as full and ordinary a life as possible.

Are there different disabilities?

There are many different kinds. In fact, this term covers such a vast range of people, with such different abilities and difficulties, that it doesn't really tell us very much. Some learning disabilities are well known and easily recognised, such as Down's syndrome. Others are more difficult to assess and diagnose, and many remain unclassified, because so little

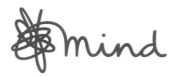

For better mental health

is known about them. In any case, it's questionable how helpful these labels are, when they can be applied to so many people with such different lives and abilities.

There are also different degrees of difficulty. At one end of the spectrum are people with very mild disabilities, who can lead ordinary lives, in jobs and relationships, with very little, if any, support. At the other end are those with very profound disabilities, who need a great deal of help to carry out everyday tasks that most of us take for granted.

What causes them?

There are many possible causes, and experts don't yet know about all of them. It's possible that there are a number of contributory factors involved at the same time. There can be something in a baby's genetic make-up that leads to complications. Sometimes, the baby doesn't develop in the usual way, either because of inheriting certain genes and chromosomes, or just by accident. The best

---

Someone who has a learning disability will have certain limitations on their ability to think (known as an impairment of intellectual ability)

---

known of these conditions is Down's syndrome, which is more common to children of older parents.

There are tests that parents may have during pregnancy, if they want to. This is a controversial issue, because many people with learning disabilities and their families feel that the idea of testing for these conditions reduces the value placed on their own lives.

Other factors during the pregnancy itself also play a part. It's thought that infections and disease, a poor diet and abusing harmful substances (such as drugs or alcohol) can affect the growing baby. Problems may also be caused by an injury to the baby before, during or after delivery. After the birth, infections such as meningitis, head injuries and extreme deprivation can sometimes be responsible.

How is it diagnosed?

Many learning disabilities are diagnosed straight after a baby has been born, or, in some cases, even beforehand, for example by an amniocentesis test during pregnancy. Health visitors and GPs are likely to pick up any undiagnosed problems (depending on their type and cause) during a baby's regular developmental checks. Most babies reach certain milestones (such as babbling, making eye contact and learning new physical skills) at around the same age. If you are concerned that your baby isn't reaching these at the right time, you should discuss this with your GP or health visitor. Sometimes, a problem isn't spotted until someone is older, when it can be diagnosed and assessed through various psychological tests.

What other problems can a learning disability bring?

It may make people more prone to certain conditions that can affect us all. For instance, it's estimated that 80 per cent of people with autism also have some level of learning disability. Epilepsy is also more common than among the rest of the population. Difficulties with communication can be another problem, particularly if a person's disability is severe.

It may be more likely for people with a learning disability to have additional physical disabilities and mental health problems. Some experts feel that it's not surprising that people are more likely to have mental health problems, given the difficulties that they face. However, the majority of people concerned don't have any additional special needs.

Prejudice and discrimination

In the past, society has often treated people with learning disabilities very badly. Misunderstanding and misinformation have kept them apart as a group. Many lived in institutions, under very poor conditions, where they were often neglected or abused.

It's not surprising that people living in these circumstances would sometimes lash out against this abusive system, but, unfortunately, this probably fed the myth that learning disabilities made people aggressive or dangerous. On the other side of this coin was the equally narrow-minded and prejudiced view that anyone with a learning disability was always child-like, happy and loving. Luckily, those days are now behind us, and people with learning disabilities are properly recognised as a diverse group of unique individuals.

The Government now actively encourages people to live in the community, so that they can stay in their own homes in their own neighbourhoods, just like anybody else. It's now accepted that everybody should have the same rights to privacy, to be treated with respect, to conduct relationships, to find meaningful work and to make choices about their everyday lives.

Unfortunately, there are still some people who feel prejudiced against people with learning disabilities, perhaps through ignorance, fear or a lack of experience. Many

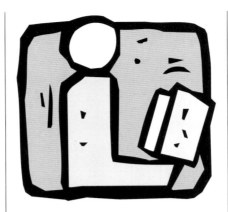

people with learning disabilities find that society's attitude towards them, and the barriers this produces, actually causes them more difficulties than their disability, although this situation should be improving, gradually.

What is it like to have a learning disability?

How we feel about ourselves is closely linked with how other people feel about us, and this is just as true for someone with a learning disability. He or she may often feel angry, sad, envious and that it's 'not fair'. These feelings are all understandable and should be acknowledged. Sometimes it's too difficult to talk about these feelings within a family and it's better to talk to a trained professional, such as a counsellor or psychotherapist.

It's important not to confuse disability with identity; your disability is not who you are. Most people learn to cope with the difficulties they face and go on to lead fulfilling lives. One way of achieving this is to accept that everyone is different and we all have things we can and can't do. By focusing on our abilities and strengths, rather than our disabilities, we are likely to have a more positive and healthy approach to life. Rather than concentrating on the fact that an individual can't talk, for example, it's better to think positively about the other ways he or she can learn to express him- or herself, such as through sign language, symbols or photographs.

What issues might parents face?

Every parent hopes for a perfect baby and, when this isn't possible, it can be a great shock and disappointment.

There are often feelings of anger, guilt and grief. If these feelings are not talked about, they can interfere with the developing bond between parents and child. For this reason, it's very important that parents get all the support, advice and counselling they need when a child is diagnosed with a disability. Talk to your GP about this, who should be able to refer you to a counsellor or psychotherapist.

Most relationships between parents and children can get quite complicated at some stage, but it's often more so when the child has a learning disability. It can be difficult for a parent to view the child as growing into an adult. Issues such as independence and sexuality are frequently very hard for parents to cope with.

While most of us learn through experience, taking risks and making mistakes, people with learning disabilities are often over-protected and denied these kinds of opportunities. Parents have the difficult task of giving their child the extra help they need, while not helping them so much they hinder them. A good approach is to think of doing everyday tasks with your child, rather than for them. When this balance is achieved it's called 'enabling'. Everybody has some level of skill that can be developed, if encouraged and nurtured.

Learning to do new things for ourselves increases our self-esteem and makes us all feel better. The learning-disabled person that is supported to be as independent as possible will be happier and more fulfilled as a result. Again, talking these issues through with a counsellor, another learning disabilities professional, or even with other parents who are in the same situation, can be very helpful.

For a catalogue of publications from Mind, send an A4 SAE to Mind Publications, 15-19 Broadway, London E15 4BQ. Tel. 0844 448 4448. Fax: 020 8534 6399. E-mail: publications@mind.org.uk

Visit the online shop to see details of all the publications stocked.

© 2004 Mind (National Association for Mental Health)

Disabled children

Information from Barnardo's

Background

In 1998 there were an estimated 393,824 disabled children under the age of 16 in the UK (three per cent of all children) and 155,976 disabled young people aged 16-19. More than 25 per cent were severely disabled, with at least two different kinds of impairment.[1]

The term 'disabled children' includes children with chronic and life-threatening or life-limiting illnesses, as well as children with learning, physical and sensory impairments, and behavioural difficulties associated with learning disabilities. Improved medical care means that more children are surviving neo-natal problems, very premature births and childhood injury. These advances, together with the closure of residential settings and long-stay hospitals during the 1980s and early 1990s, means that there are more disabled children now living in the community, many of whom have very complex care needs.

The 'social' and 'medical' models of disability

Disability is commonly seen as a problem which an individual has, but in recent years disabled people have taken the view that while they may have functional limitations of mind or body, these impairments in themselves do not prevent them from living ordinary lives.

In many cases, it is the barriers in everyday life which cause the disability. For instance, wheelchair users may be denied opportunities because the places they wish to go are inaccessible, or people with learning disabilities may fail at tasks they have the potential to perform because they do not get the right training.

One in 10 citizens of the European Union is disabled in some way, and seven out of 10 develop impairment during their lifetime,[2] yet our buildings, vehicles, education system, health care services, leisure

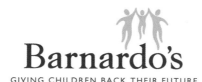

Barnardo's
GIVING CHILDREN BACK THEIR FUTURE

facilities and employment structures are not designed to take account of people's differences.

The 'medical' model of disability tends to focus on the physical, sensory or intellectual impairment of the person as the problem. This has in the past contributed to the exclusion of disabled people from mainstream economic and social activity.

The 'social' model of disability sees disability as a result of society's failure to adapt to the needs arising from a person's medical condition. It aims to identify and tackle the disabling barriers which prevent people with impairments from leading normal lives. Impairment – the functional limitations of someone's mind or body – is separated from disability, which is caused by prejudice and unequal access to education, employment, housing, transport and leisure activities.

A good education is important for all young people, but particularly for those facing disadvantage, such as disabled children

---

Barnardo's believes that society's failure to adapt to allow disabled children and young people the same level of access and opportunity as non-disabled children is a breach of their human rights.

Education

One of the most important ways in which disabled children are excluded from society at an early age is through the education system. A good education is important for all young people, but particularly for those facing disadvantage, such as disabled children. An incomplete or sub-standard education means fewer job opportunities and less chance of becoming independent.

There is still a common perception that disabled children cannot be adequately catered for in the mainstream, and that they require separate schooling. Catchment areas for special schools can be very wide and many LEAs transport their children over long distances on the grounds that they cannot meet their needs locally. This isolates children from their communities and forces them to spend hours travelling to and from school each day.

Segregated education and a lack of everyday interaction with disabled people help to perpetuate misunderstanding and discrimination among non-disabled people. The evidence suggests that children with a range of impairments, including those who have learning, behavioural or cognitive difficulties, do better in an inclusive rather than special educational setting. However, their performance may be compromised in school settings which do not value and promote a co-operative learning style. In particular, the psycho-social development of disabled children in inclusive settings may suffer in comparison to that of children in special education if insufficient attention is paid to their support needs.[2]

Children educated outside the mainstream tend to achieve less academically, have less confidence and self-esteem, and are ill-prepared for adult life. The choices for disabled young people about further education or work in adulthood are often very limited, and many face long-term dependence on the social security system, or adult forms of residential provision.

The Special Educational Needs and Disability Act (Senda) 2002 strengthens the right of disabled children to a place in mainstream school and requires schools to make 'reasonable' adjustments to become accessible and enable disabled children to participate in the curriculum and other aspects of school life. Progress is likely to be incremental and it may be some time before disabled children routinely go to their local school. Achieving this will require considerable will and effort from parents, local authorities and schools – plus the resources – to make it happen. Some local authorities have already demonstrated a commitment to inclusive education, and Senda will further promote this.

What is inclusion?

Inclusion is a concept which involves the adaptation of all parts of the community – both in people's attitudes and the physical environment – to cater for a wide spectrum of ability and need. This needs to be an ongoing process, the overall aim of which is to embrace diversity rather than simply tolerate differences.

The Disability Discrimination Act 1995 laid down rights for disabled people to have the same access to 'goods and services' as other members of the public. Senda also requires schools and youth services to make 'reasonable adjustments' to ensure that disabled pupils are not disadvantaged.

But inclusion means more than providing physical access to buildings and facilities – important as this is. To be inclusive, both institutions and the people in them need to change and develop. The terms 'integration' and 'inclusion' are often used interchangeably, but they have different meanings. When a child is integrated, there may be specialist support available, but the child has to fit in with the existing system. An inclusive system sees diversity as positive and is responsive to this, rather than trying to make everyone fit a pre-determined structure.

Making inclusion work

Inclusion can only be successful with appropriate resources and planning – it cannot be achieved simply by placing disabled children in mainstream settings. Physical access to buildings and facilities is very important, but inclusion also means offering services tailored to individual needs, which provide a real choice and enable young people to succeed. Services must meet the needs of children at different ages and stages, and take into account the fact that some children need very specialised support. It is important too that disabled children have opportunities to network with other disabled children.

Making the transition to fully inclusive communities and services requires the redeployment of resources and facilities over a period of time. Inclusion should not be seen as a cheap option, and cannot be achieved without adequate funding and resources. However, the Audit Commission found that educating a child with learning disabilities in a mainstream school with the right support was no more expensive than a place in a special school.[3]

Most importantly, inclusion is about challenging and changing commonly held attitudes towards disabled people and promoting their right to participate as fully in life as others. Many of the changes necessary to achieve inclusion – to attitudes, systems and environments – will only take place as disabled people become more involved in the mainstream and in making their views, needs and experiences felt.

■ Barnardo's believes that every child, whatever their needs, has the right to participate fully in their community and to have the same choices, opportunities and experiences as other children. To achieve this for disabled children, there needs to be the right kind of support and a willingness to adapt on the part of everyone in society.

References
1 NCH (2002), *NCH Factfile 2002-2003*
2 Commission of the European Communities (1996), *Helios II European Guide of Good Practice Towards Equal Opportunities for Disabled People*, Office for Official Publications of the European Communities.
3 Peetsma, T.; Vergeer, M.; Roeleveld, J.; Karsten, S. (2001) Inclusion in Education: comparing pupils' development in special and regular education. *Educational Review*, 2001, vol. 53, no. 2, pp. 125-136
4 Audit Commission (1992), *Getting in on the Act*, Stationery Office

■ The above information is from Barnardo's. For more information visit their website which can be found at www.barnardos.org.uk

© *Barnardo's*

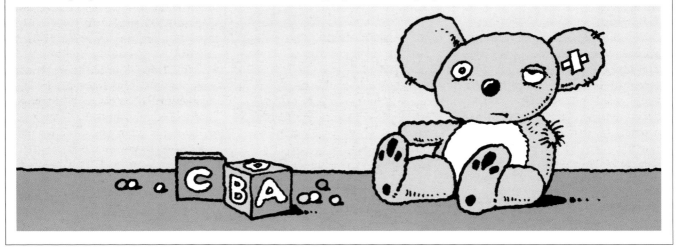

Living with the education system

The experiences of people with a learning disability

Children and adults with a learning disability have widely varying experiences of school and college. Here are some examples of the difficulties and successes that people have experienced:

Anna's story

Anna is six years old. She has a rare syndrome that results in a moderate learning disability, poor muscle tone and speech and language difficulties.

Anna attends a small voluntary-aided school and is supported by a teaching assistant for ten hours each week. Some of this support is during class time and the rest during breaks. At lunchtime, her assistant runs a physical activity group for a small group of pupils.

Before Anna attended the school, it had very little experience of special educational needs, let alone such complex needs. It was the leadership of the head teacher that made the situation work. She supported Anna's parents and applied to the local education authority to get the resources the school needed. With Mencap and Anna's mother, the head teacher devised a series of short training events, which helped all the staff become much more confident when working with Anna.

David's story

David wanted to go on a school trip to an Outward Bound centre. At first the school said that it would be inappropriate for him to go as he has a learning disability. They insisted that he would not have been able to stay in the same room as other pupils in case he became ill and had an epileptic fit. The school also said that David's mother would have had to accompany him on the trip to administer medication, as they could not arrange alternative support.

After David's family complained, the school recognised that it could not exclude David from the school trip. But instead of providing health support for David, they decided to cancel all future school trips for him and his classmates.

Rachel's story

Rachel is 15 and has Down's syndrome. She went to her local primary school, where she was in a special needs class. When she left primary school, she and her parents wanted her to go to the local middle school with her elder brother. The local education authority (LEA) said that she ought to go to a special school 15 miles away. One of the officials in the LEA said: 'She'll be the thickest child in the school. Do you think she'll cope with that?'

Rachel's parents refused to accept that a special school was the right answer. They pursued every avenue they could to enable her to go to school with her brother, and got the help of local support groups. Finally the LEA backed down and Rachel went to the school she wanted.

A couple of years ago, Rachel transferred to a local high school

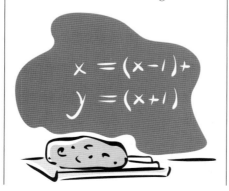

that has a strong special educational needs team and a head teacher who is committed to inclusion. He said: 'It's Rachel's right to come here. We want to have her.'

Rachel's mother has no doubts about having fought so hard to get Rachel into local mainstream schools. She says: 'If Rachel had gone to special school 15 miles away, I don't believe she would be the young person she is today. She has lots of friends locally and is part of the community. That's what we wanted for her.'

Special Educational Needs and Disability Act

Mencap has helped to ensure that the Special Educational Needs and Disability Act, which became law in April 2001, considers the needs of children with a learning disability.

This Act makes it unlawful to discriminate on the grounds of disability in schools and colleges, and strengthens the rights of children with special educational needs.

Mencap did a lot of work to ensure this law really helps children with a learning disability. It lobbied MPs and peers, and also chaired the parliamentary group of the Special Educational Consortium. This group brought together more than 200 charities representing the interests of children with special needs. Mencap's key aims were:

- to support the Government in bringing disability rights into education to make sure that schools and colleges plan to support pupils with a learning disability.
- The lobbying gained a lot of changes to the Act.

■ The above information is from Mencap's website which can be found at www.mencap.org.uk

© Mencap

Is disability a barrier to working in education?

Inclusive education does not only mean the integration of disabled children into mainstream schools – it also refers to teaching staff

Mainstreaming in many countries now means that disabled children aren't uncommon in today's schools. But it's still considered unusual for a disabled person to be at the front of the classroom.

A recent study completed at the University of Wales (UWCN) in the United Kingdom has prompted widespread debate as to why very few young disabled people are choosing a career in teaching. The report, issued by the UWCN's School of Education, highlights 'prejudice and ignorance' as the two main contributing factors.

But this problem is not unique to the UK. Despite a global shortage of qualified teaching staff, many education authorities are reluctant to employ disabled teachers because of their own perceived stereotypes of what disabled people are capable of.

Another issue is lack of role models. As with all professions, role models are needed for children and young adults to aspire to. The lack of disabled teachers currently working in education is another reason why young disabled people are not choosing teaching as a career.

Teacher prejudices

Of course, there is also the global issue of poor remuneration and working conditions, which affects all teachers. The shortage of funds available to make the necessary reforms in order to accommodate disabled students and disabled staff is another major contributing factor. While many educational authorities are required by law to cater for the educational needs of disabled students, very little funding or attention is given to the needs of disabled teaching staff.

Classroom style

There are also too many instances

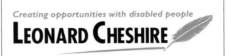

Creating opportunities with disabled people
LEONARD CHESHIRE

when disabled people who do teach or want to become teachers face barriers and prejudice.

David was diagnosed with multiple sclerosis 15 years ago and was a special education teacher in Montreal, Canada, until recently, when, in the face of continued discrimination from his employers, he was forced to resign. Rather than focusing on his experience, skill and popularity in the classroom, the administration chose to highlight the more negative aspects of his performance such as his rare absences due to illness and his reluctance to teach a group of 24 children with special needs in a classroom which did not adequately meet their or his needs. David is currently taking legal action against his dismissal.

There are also more positive examples of disabled people who pursue a successful career in the classroom. Sally, from Northampton, England, is spending the summer preparing her classrooms for the new school year. She has put up calendars, posters and alphabet charts on the freshly painted walls but perhaps most critically she has arranged the furniture. Sally teaches from a wheelchair and so has to make sure that there is adequate space to

---

Despite a global shortage of qualified teaching staff, many education authorities are reluctant to employ disabled teachers

---

manoeuvre around the desks and chairs. 'Clearly there are challenges to overcome, both for me and my employer. But neither has let my disability get in the way.

'Too many people with disabilities have spent their lives listening to people telling them what they can't do instead of what they can. Consequently, I am very open about my disability and answer every, well nearly every, question thrown at me about it.'

New role models

So why employ disabled teachers? Once employed, disabled staff can make an important contribution to the overall school curriculum, as effective employees, in raising the aspirations of disabled students and increasing the awareness of disability throughout the school community. And when schools employ disabled teachers effectively, it is likely to improve their ability to meet other fundamental social and legal requirements. For instance, a building that's accessible to a teacher who uses a wheelchair should have ramps, lift access and wide doorways, so it will also be accessible to students and parents with similar needs. But perhaps one of the most important reasons is that a disabled teacher can provide an essential role model for disabled students, providing evidence that this profession is open to them.

Compass has found that there are currently no accurate statistics detailing the number of disabled teachers employed in the UK and Canada.

■ The above information is from the Leonard Cheshire magazine *Compass*. For more information visit their website which can be found at www.leonard-cheshire.org

© *Leonard Cheshire*

Left holding the baby

Discriminatory attitudes mean people with learning disabilities get a raw deal at the hands of the NHS, says a new report. By Debbie Andalo and Alison Benjamin

Frances Affleck worried that if she ever became a parent, there was no guarantee that the doctor would have the skills or the patience to explain to her clearly how her baby was developing and what to do if it had colic or a common cold. Affleck, 29, knew the NHS had neither the time nor the skills to help adults who, like her, are diagnosed with learning disabilities.

But now she hopes new parents will be able to help themselves with the publication of her book, *You and Your Baby 0-1*, which will steer parents through the first year of their baby's life. Using pictures with simple words, there is advice about common baby health problems, child development and how to breast feed, as well as pictures which help explain the roles of different health professionals.

Affleck, who is a project worker for the disability rights organisation Change, says: 'This is the book I would want to read if I ever had a baby. If parents with learning disabilities don't have access to health information like this, they feel frustrated and upset.'

The book, funded by the Department for Education and Skills, was due to be published in July 2004. At the same time, Change is producing a 'health picture bank' CD aimed at health professionals that includes 500 pictures they can use to help explain clinical issues to patients with learning disabilities.

Philipa Bragman, Change director, says: 'We are trying to provide the tools to make the health service more accessible to people with learning difficulties. The pictures tell the story, and because they have been compiled by people who have learning disabilities, they should be able to get over a sense of what is going on.'

The exclusion that people with learning difficulties feel from the health service was highlighted in June 2004 by disability charity Mencap, which commissioned a survey that showed 70% of GP surgeries have no information that those with learning disabilities can easily understand. Moreover, 75% of family doctors say they have received no training to help them treat people with a learning disability, and 80% thought the Department of Health should provide medical students and practitioners with more training. Nine in 10 admitted a patient's learning disability had made it more difficult to give a diagnosis.

Assumptions and value judgements made by healthcare professionals are a barrier to people with learning disabilities receiving a correct diagnosis and accessing appropriate care

---

A GP with a list of 2,000 patients is estimated to have about 40 patients with a learning disability, of which about eight will have severe problems. Epilepsy, dementia, schizophrenia, and thyroid problems are some of the medical conditions that people with a learning disability are more at risk from than the rest of the population.

The survey of 215 GPs is contained in a report by Mencap that highlights how assumptions and value judgements made by healthcare professionals are a barrier to people with learning disabilities receiving a correct diagnosis and accessing appropriate care. Hospital practice fares as badly as primary care. While hospitals have a statutory duty to care for all patients, the report, *Treat Me Right!*, raises concerns about how negative or discriminatory attitudes and poor communication skills among healthcare staff can con-tribute to people with learning disabilities being much more likely to die before the age of 50 – often from respiratory problems or coronary heart disease.

Katherine was only 30 when she went into hospital suffering from chest problems. When she was put on an intravenous drip, the hospital staff forgot to include her epilepsy medication in the drip feed. As a result, she had a violent and prolonged fit and died.

Max was 30 when he fell and broke his hip. What should have been a routine operation resulted in his death a few weeks later because no one noticed he had developed a kidney problem and become mal-nourished.

'We were really shocked by the number of premature deaths we uncovered,' says David Congdon, Mencap's head of external relations. 'While everyone understands that anyone can get cancer or have a major heart attack, people like Max should never have died. There are many stories of parents feeling obliged to stay with their child in hospital because of fears that they will be neglected or denied treatment. When something goes wrong we don't know if it's because of poor care that anyone could have received, or if it is discriminatory. We have suspicions but it is very difficult to prove.'

In 2001, a report published into allegations made against the Royal Brompton and Harefield Hospitals, that children were refused heart surgery because they had Down's syndrome, upheld claims that doctors had failed to provide a 'balanced view' of the treatment options available.

The Mencap report calls on government to set up a confidential inquiry into mortality among people with learning difficulties. 'It is the only way to discover whether there is a systemic problem in the service,' says Congdon. 'It would also answer questions such as "how many people a year with a learning disability die prematurely?" No figures exist.' The report recommends that the government should fund GPs to carry out voluntary annual health checks for people with a learning disability, so that signs and symptoms of ill health can be diagnosed earlier.

The Department of Health did recognise in its learning disability white paper, *Valuing People*, 2001, that the quality of healthcare was 'too variable'. It points to good practice guidance issued in July 2002 on two key elements of its strategy to improve the health of people with learning disabilities: health action plans and health facilitation.

Later this year, it expects to bring forward proposals to offer disabled people the option of an annual health check, but has no plans to launch a confidential inquiry into

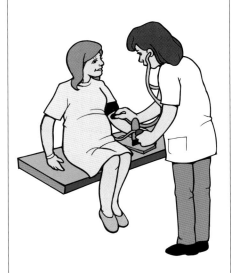

premature deaths. 'At present we aim to use funds to concentrate on health action planning and other related activity, that will help to bring better health to people with learning disabilities in the short term,' says a DoH spokeswoman.

Earlier this month, it also set up a disability access working group, with the Disability Rights Commission, to develop initiatives to improve access to information and services for people with any disability, as well as raising awareness of disability issues among healthcare professionals.

But Mencap accuses the government of 'ducking the issue'. 'They'll only get to the root of the problem by investigating if there is a systemic problem,' says Congdon. 'Mencap will have no option but to back parents of children with a learning disability who want to take individual legal action when they suspect there has been discrimination in the health service.'

■ For more information about *You and Your Baby 0-1* or the CD, contact Change at www.changepeople.co.uk

© *Guardian Newspapers Limited 2004*

Call for more support for older carers

By Alison Benjamin

Organisations set up to support people with learning disabilities are failing older families, according to a report.

It reveals that fewer than 40% of partnership boards are helping people with learning disabilities with older family carers plan for their future needs.

The report, *Planning for Tomorrow*, by the Foundation for People with Learning Disabilities (FPLD), says less than half of boards know how many people with learning disabilities live at home with a family carer aged 70 or over.

The findings come from a survey of 70 partnership boards across England. Respondents reported a lack of resources and capacity to meet priorities for supporting older family carers.

The government's *Valuing People* white paper on learning disability estimates that a third of people with learning disabilities living in the family home are cared for by a relative aged 70 or over.

It recognises that lack of planning for the future creates anxiety and stress for the whole family and sets targets for local partnership boards to support these older families which include identifying carers aged over 70 and prioritising this group for person-centred planning.

But the survey shows that processes for monitoring the needs of older family carers tend to be 'ad-hoc and generally poor'.

Hazel Morgan, head of FPLD, says partnership boards must employ dedicated workers and monitor older family carers regularly. '[This] can only be resourced with long-term funding commitments,' she says.

Planning for Tomorrow recommends that the Department of Health ring-fence money from the learning disability development fund and carers' grant.

It also identifies a clear need for learning disability services to make stronger links with older people's social and primary health care services to provide a more 'joined up' approach to supporting older family carers.

Ms Morgan urges partnership boards to go beyond government targets and start planning for when younger carers reach 60 in order to avoid unnecessary crises.

The report is part of the older families' carers' initiative, a three-year project funded by the DoH and led by the FPLD. It is designed to support partnership boards across England to identify and meet the needs of older family carers of people with learning disabilities.

■ *Planning for Tomorrow* is available at £10.

© *Guardian Newspapers Limited 2004*

When health for all doesn't mean all

Providing all patients with greater choice and tackling growing obesity levels are just two of the ways in which the Government is trying to improve the general health of the nation. But as Mencap's latest campaign, being launched during Learning Disability Week, aims to highlight, people with a learning disability are still getting the worst deal when it comes to accessing health care. By David Congdon, Head of External Relations

It is a fundamental human right that all people should get good quality health care. People with a learning disability generally have worse health than others and often this is a result of poor health care. The sad reality is that many people with a learning disability die at an unnecessarily young age. It is this quite unacceptable fact which has prompted Mencap to launch the *Treat me right!* campaign.

During Learning Disability Week (held from 21-27 June 2004), Mencap published a report to kick-start the campaign. *Treat me right!* highlights the health care concerns and experiences of people with a learning disability across the country. One of its key aims will be to increase levels of awareness and understanding among health professionals and others working with people with a learning disability.

Research on the health of people with a learning disability is compelling. People with a learning disability are:

- three times more likely to die from respiratory disease;
- at greater risk of coronary heart disease, making this the second most common cause of death (14-20%);
- more likely to get gastrointestinal cancer and stomach disorders.

Certainly, the facts are startling but they do not fully explain the high number of early deaths.

People with a learning disability are of course more likely to have certain health problems, such as epilepsy and sight and hearing impairments, which are related to their disability. But this must not be used as an excuse for failing to tackle a fundamental problem: people with a learning disability have poor experiences of using health services and this has a bad effect on their health.

One of the main problems is around good communications. Medical and nursing staff need to be able to understand what it means to have a learning disability and how to recognise their special needs. A lot of this is about changing attitudes.

There is also a major problem with what is known as 'diagnostic over-shadowing'. This is where doctors will look at someone with a learning disability and consciously or unconsciously believe that their health problem is the result of a learning disability and that not much can be done about it. The danger of this is that it can lead to undiagnosed or misdiagnosed conditions. This has recently been highlighted by the National Patient Safety Agency.

Medical and nursing staff need to be able to understand what it means to have a learning disability and how to recognise their special needs

---

Poor care in hospitals is another long-standing issue. This often results in hospitals expecting parents and carers to help feed or care for their son or daughter. There have been cases of people with a learning disability being neglected in hospital because they are unable to tell staff they are in pain or that something has gone wrong with their intravenous drip.

Treat me right! is a wake-up call to the health service to take this issue seriously. Over many years, despite good government policy and guidance, nothing much has changed. In June, Mencap will be making a number of key recommendations aimed mainly at Primary Care Trusts in England and their equivalents in Wales and Northern Ireland. These will include annual health checks to be offered to all people with a learning disability, better learning disability training for all healthcare staff, and accessible information to be provided in all GP surgeries and other healthcare settings.

- For more information about the *Treat me right!* campaign, go to: www.mencap.org.uk/treatmeright

For information on other events and activities taking place during Learning Disability Week, go to: www.mencap.org.uk/ldw

Key points

- During Learning Disability Week in June, Mencap will launch its *Treat me right!* campaign.
- This will look at the unequal treatment of people with a learning disability in GP surgeries and hospitals.
- Mencap will explain what needs to be done to make sure people with a learning disability get equal access to healthcare. It will also highlight good and bad practice.

- The above information is from *Viewpoint* May/June 2004, the magazine produced by Mencap.

© *Mencap*

- In general, the attitudes of the British public towards disability and disabled people are broadly positive and supportive. (p. 2)

- Slightly higher proportions of boys (19 per cent) than girls (17 per cent) aged under 20 years reported having a mild disability in 2000. Rates of severe disability were consistently higher for boys than girls with 11 per 10,000 of the male population and five per 10,000 of the female population aged under 17 years in 2000. (p. 4)

- Disabled people continue to face discrimination and difficulties imposed by society in every area of their lives. (p. 6)

- Of those looking for work, disabled people made an average of two and a half times as many job applications as non-disabled people and yet got fewer job offers. (p. 7)

- Around 10 million people are affected by disability including almost 20% of the UK working-age population. (p. 9)

- In October 2004 the provisions of the Disability Discrimination Act (DDA) will be extended to include employers with two or more employees. This will greatly increase the percentage of employers covered by the provisions of the DDA. (p. 10)

- People who have a disability as defined, who believe they have been the subject of discrimination in employment matters or consider a reasonable adjustment has not been made, may complain to an employment tribunal. (p. 12)

- The Disability Discrimination Act extends to firms employing fewer than 15 staff in October and requires all businesses to provide equal physical access to their products and services or face the threat of prosecution. (p. 15)

- Firms have been banned since 1999 from enforcing policies that prevent disabled customers using their services. (p. 16)

- The Government has published the Children Bill which is now going through Parliament. Mencap is concerned that the Bill does not contain enough about disabled children. (p. 18)

- Disabled employees have the same aspirations and ambitions as anyone else in the workforce. They want jobs which are challenging and rewarding and are just as likely to want opportunities for career development and promotion. (p. 20)

- 87 per cent of people questioned by YouGov said that disabled people should have equal rights with non-disabled people and 40 per cent felt there aren't enough disabled people on television. (p. 22)

- Despite the UK's Government manifesto commitment in 2001 to implement all the Disability Rights Taskforce's outstanding recommendations relating to transport, there is a continued failure to do. Today eight and a half million – or one in seven of the UK population – are still struggling to get on board. (p. 25)

- The formal definition of 'learning disabilities' or 'intellectual disabilities' includes the presence of:
  – a significant intellectual impairment and
  – deficits in social functioning or adaptive behaviour
  – which are present from childhood. (p. 26)

- Approximately £4.6 billion is spent a year to provide formal services for children and adults with learning disabilities in the UK. (p. 26)

- Many learning disabilities are diagnosed straight after a baby has been born, or, in some cases, even beforehand, for example by an amniocentesis test during pregnancy. (p. 27)

- A good education is important for all young people, but particularly for those facing disadvantage, such as disabled children. (p. 29)

- Mencap has helped to ensure that the Special Educational Needs and Disability Act, which became law in April 2001, considers the needs of children with a learning disability. This Act makes it unlawful to discriminate on the grounds of disability in schools and colleges, and strengthens the rights of children with special educational needs. (p. 31)

- Despite a global shortage of qualified teaching staff, many education authorities are reluctant to employ disabled teachers. (p. 32)

- Assumptions and value judgements made by healthcare professionals are a barrier to people with learning disabilities receiving a correct diagnosis and accessing appropriate care. (p. 37)

- The government's Valuing People white paper on learning disability estimates that a third of people with learning disabilities living in the family home are cared for by a relative aged 70 or over. (p. 38)

- Medical and nursing staff need to be able to understand what it means to have a learning disability and how to recognise their special needs. (p. 39)

ADDITIONAL RESOURCES

You might like to contact the following organisations for further information. Due to the increasing cost of postage, many organisations cannot respond to enquiries unless they receive a stamped, addressed envelope.

Ability Media Ltd
Business & Innovation Centre
Sunderland Enterprise Park
Sunderland
Tyne & Wear, SR5 2TA
Tel: 0845 456 1091
Fax: 0191 516 6849
E-mail: info@ukability.co.uk
Website: www.ukability.co.uk/index.html
Provides a disability information resource that is comprehensive, useful, and ultimately accessible to everyone.

Advisory, Conciliation & Arbitration Service (ACAS)
Brandon House
180 Borough High Street
London, SE1 1LW
Tel: 020 7210 3613
Website: www.acas.org.uk
Aims to improve organisations and working life through better employment relations.

Barnardo's
Tanners Lane
Barkingside
Ilford, Essex, IG6 1QG
Tel: 020 8550 8822
Fax: 020 8551 6870
Website: www.barnardos.org.uk
Barnardo's works with over 47,000 children, young people and their families in more than 300 projects across the county including work with children affected by today's most urgent issues; homelessness, poverty, disability and abuse.

Disability Rights Commission (DRC)
222 Grays Inn Road
London, WC1X 8HL
Tel: 020 754 37000
E-mail: info@drc-gb.org
Website: www.drc-gb.org
The Disability Rights Commission (DRC) has been set up to promote civil rights for disabled people.

The Employers' Forum on Disability
Nutmeg House
60 Gainsford Street
London, SE1 2NY
Tel: 020 7403 3020
Fax: 020 7403 0404
Website: www.employers-forum.co.uk
The national employers' organisation focused on disability in the UK.

The Foundation for People with Learning Disabilities
83 Victoria Street
London, SW1H OHW
Tel: 020 7802 0300
Fax: 020 7802 0301
E-mail: fpld@fpld.org.uk
Website: www.learningdisabilities.org.uk
Works with people with learning disabilities to improve the quality of their lives.

Leonard Cheshire
Leonard Cheshire House
30 Millbank
London, SW1P 4QD
Tel: 020 7802 8200
Fax: 020 7802 8250
E-mail: info@london.leonard-cheshire.org.uk
Website: www.leonard-cheshire.org
Provides a range of care services for people with physical or learning disabilities and those with mental health problems.

Mencap
123 Golden Lane
London, EC1Y 0RT
Tel: 020 7454 0454
Fax: 020 7608 3254
E-mail: help@mencap.org.uk
Website: www.mencap.org.uk
Mencap is the UK's leading learning disability charity working with people with a learning disability and their families and carers.

Mind (National Association for Mental Health)
Granta House, 15-19 Broadway
Stratford, London, E15 4BQ
Tel: 020 8519 2122
Fax: 020 8522 1725
E-mail: contact@mind.org.uk
Website: www.mind.org.uk
Mind works for a better life for everyone with experience of mental distress.

RADAR
12 City Forum, 250 City Road
London, EC1V 8AF
Tel: 020 7250 3222
Fax: 020 7250 0212
E-mail: radar@radar.org.uk
Website: www.radar.org.uk
RADAR's vision is of a society where human difference is routinely anticipated, expertly accommodated and positively celebrated.

Scope
6-10 Market Road
London, N7 9PW
Tel: 020 7619 7100
Fax: 020 7436 2601
Website: www.scope.org.uk
The disability organisation in England and Wales whose focus is people with cerebral palsy. Their aim is that disabled people achieve equality: a society in which they are as valued and have the same human and civil rights as everyone else.

Skill: National Bureau for Students with Disabililties
Chapter House
18-20 Crucifix Lane
London, SE1 3JW
Tel: 020 7450 0620
Fax: 020 7450 0650
E-mail: admin@skill.org.uk
Website: www.skill.org.uk
Skill is a national charity promoting opportunities for young people and adults with any kind of disability in post-16 education, training and employment across the UK.

INDEX

horseriding 4
housing 11
    rented housing 17

I

identity 28
inclusion concept 29-30, 30, 32
independent living 11
information provision 11, 12
Into Higher Education 35

L

landlords 17
language to describe disability 6
learning disabilities 26-39
    autistic spectrum disorders 26, 28
    and bullying 26
    carers' needs 38
    causes of 26, 27
    children with 28, 29-30
    definition 26, 27
    diagnosing 27
    and health care 37-8, 39
    and identity 28
    inclusion concept 30, 32
    and mental health 4, 26
    number of people with 26, 29
    types of 27
    see also education
Learning Disability Week 39
legislation 17
    Children Bill 18
    Special Educational Needs and Disability Act (2001) 7, 10, 30, 31
    see also Disability Discrimination Act
Leonard Cheshire Foundation 5, 6, 25, 32
Lifetime Homes standards 11
listed buildings 15
London Underground 25

M

manufactured goods 13
medical model of disability 6, 29
MENCAP 31, 37, 39
mental handicaps see learning disabilities
MIND 27-8
mobility disability 1
models of disability 6, 29

N

NHS (National Health Service) 11, 37-8
numbers of disabled people 4, 6, 14

O

The Office 23

P

parenthood 3
parking spaces 2, 10
paying extra for rights of disabled people 3
Pennington, Sara 33-4

physical features adjustments 13, 14
Planning for Tomorrow 38
polling stations 6
poverty 9
Prime Minister's Strategy Unit 9
public attitudes to disability 2-4
public transport *see* transport standards
purchasing power of disabled people 14

Q

quality of life 9

R

RADAR 10-11
rates of disability *see* numbers of disabled people
reasonable adjustment duty 12, 30
rented housing 17
retardation *see* learning disabilities
Rhead, Sarah-Jane 35
Rickell, Andy 5
Ripple school 33-4
Roberts, Andy 34
Rotinsulu, Maulani 5

S

Scarlet, Mick 23
Scope 2-4, 6-8, 22
SEN Statements 7, 34
service and goods provision 7, 8, 13-14
shops 15
smaller companies 15-16
Smith, Colin 15
Smith, Ricky 33
social model of disability 6, 29
Spanton, Viv 25
Special Educational Needs and Disability Act (2001) 7, 10, 30, 31
sports clubs 17
students 35
    graduate recruitment 19-20
    wheelchair students 36
swimming 4

T

teaching careers 32
teenagers, rates of disability 4
television 21-2, 23-4
transport standards 8, 10, 17, 25
tribunal claims 12
Tyler, Richard 15-16

U

UBS 20

W

wheelchair students 36
Whizz-Kidz 21-2
workplace alterations 15-16

Y

YouGov survey 2-4, 22

ACKNOWLEDGEMENTS

The publisher is grateful for permission to reproduce the following material.

While every care has been taken to trace and acknowledge copyright, the publisher tenders its apology for any accidental infringement or where copyright has proved untraceable. The publisher would be pleased to come to a suitable arrangement in any such case with the rightful owner.

Overview
Definition of disability, © 2004 Disability Rights Commission, *Public attitudes to disabilities*, © YouGov, *Knowledge of famous disabled people*, © YouGov, *Disability*, © Crown copyright is reproduced with the permission of Her Majesty's Stationery Office, *Young people with disabilities*, © Crown copyright is reproduced with the permission of Her Majesty's Stationery Office, *World of their own?*, © Leonard Cheshire, *Disability issues*, © Scope, *Action needed to improve disabled people's lives*, © Crown copyright is reproduced with the permission of Her Majesty's Stationery Office, *Disability Living Allowance*, © Crown copyright is reproduced with the permission of Her Majesty's Stationery Office, *Still itching for change*, © RADAR, *Economic activity*, © Crown copyright is reproduced with the permission of Her Majesty's Stationery Office.

Chapter One: Discrimination
Disability discrimination, © Advisory, Conciliation and Arbitration Service (Acas), *Open 4 all*, © 2004 Disability Rights Commission, *Disability in the UK*, © Employers' Forum on Disability 2004, *How to get in on the Disability Act*, © Telegraph Group Limited, London 2004, *Single body will cover all acts of discrimination*, © Telegraph Group Limited, London 2004, *Making new laws to protect disabled people*, © Crown copyright is reproduced with the permission of Her Majesty's Stationery Office, *Disabled children left out in the cold again?*, © Mencap, *To be or not to be honest?*, © Kate Crockett, *Disabled people as workers*, © Employers' Forum on Disability 2004, *Disability on TV*, © 2004 Whizz-Kidz, *Disablism*, © Scope, *Serious about laughter*, © Ability Media Ltd, *Public transport?*, © Leonard Cheshire.

Chapter Two: Learning Disabilities
Statistics on learning disabilities, © Foundation for People with Learning Disabilities, *Understanding learning disabilities*, © Mind (National Association for Mental Health), *Disabled children*, © Barnardo's, *Living with the education system*, © Mencap, *Is disability a barrier to working in education?*, © Leonard Cheshire, *Mainstream but special*, © Sara Pennington, *Special Educational Needs (SEN)*, © Crown copyright is reproduced with the permission of Her Majesty's Stationery Office, *Legal rights for disabled students*, © Skill: National Bureau for Students with Disabilities, *Ruling forces college to accept wheelchair student*, © Telegraph Group Limited, London 2004, *Left holding the baby*, © Guardian Newspapers Limited 2004, *Call for more support for older carers*, © Guardian Newspapers Limited 2004, *When health for all doesn't mean all*, © Mencap.

Photographs and illustrations:
Pages 1, 18, 23, 33, 36: Simon Kneebone; pages 6, 26: Angelo Madrid; pages 12, 21: Bev Aisbett; pages 15, 25: Pumpkin House; pages 17, 30, 35: Don Hatcher.

Craig Donnellan
Cambridge
September, 2004